Insomnia
A Clinical Guide to Assessment and Treatment

Insomnia
A Clinical Guide to Assessment and Treatment

Charles M. Morin
Université Laval
Quebec, Canada

and

Colin A. Espie
University of Glasgow
Glasgow, Scotland

Kluwer Academic / Plenum Publishers
New York   Boston   Dordrecht   London   Moscow

Library of Congress Cataloging-in-Publication Data

Insomnia: a clinical guide to assessment and treatment/edited by Charles M. Morin and
Colin A. Espie.
    p.   cm.
    Includes bibliographical references and index.
    ISBN 0-306-47750-5
      1. Insomnia. I. Morin, Charles M. II. Espie, Colin A.
    [DNLM: 1. Sleep Initiation and Maintenance Disorders—diagnosis. 2. Sleep Initiation
and Maintenance Disorders—therapy. WM 188 I589 2003]
    RC548.I557 2003
    616.8′498—dc21

                                     2003051325

ISBN 0-306-47750-5

©2003 Kluwer Academic / Plenum Publishers, New York
233 Spring Street, New York, New York 10013

http://www.wkap.nl/

10 9 8 7 6 5 4 3 2 1

A C.I.P. record for this book is available from the Library of Congress

Permissions for books published in Europe: *permissions@wkap.nl*
Permissions for books published in the United States of America: *permissions@wkap.com*

Printed in the United States of America

*To our children, Geneviève and Sébastien (CM) and Craig,
Carolyn, and Robbie (CE), for their love and inspiration,
and to Rena whose courage in adversity is
an example to follow (CE)*

Preface

Along with increasing recognition of the consequences and costs of insomnia, there is growing evidence documenting the effectiveness of cognitive-behavior therapy for insomnia. Yet, there is still a major gap between available evidence and current clinical practice. Much of this gap is due to economics, limited treatment access, and ineffective dissemination of knowledge. There is a definite need for practical materials to facilitate access to and implementation of interventions for insomnia. As scientists-practitioners, we are constantly reminded of this need by frequent requests from clinicians around the world for questionnaires and handouts to assist them in treating insomnia patients. It was during a recent international sleep meeting, more specifically on a train journey between Dresden and Prague, that we drafted an outline of a handbook that would help fill this gap.

This clinical handbook describes an evidence-based treatment program for insomnia. Its content is based on materials that have been clinically tested and validated with patients in various settings and with different subtypes of insomnia. The manual is divided into eight chapters. Chapter 1 presents an introduction to sleep and provides answers to frequently asked questions about the nature of sleep, its determinants, and about the consequences of sleep loss and insomnia. Chapters 2 and 3 outline the main clinical features of insomnia and differential diagnostic issues and describe a practical approach to the assessment of insomnia complaint. Chapters 4–6 provide a step-by-step description of the treatment program, including sleep hygiene guidelines, relaxation therapy, behavioral and sleep scheduling strategies, and cognitive interventions. Chapter 7 covers the essentials of sleep medications, their indications, risks and benefits, as well as clinical guidelines to discontinue their usage among prolonged users. Chapter 8 concludes with practical strategies for effective treatment implementation and addresses clinical issues arising when working with older adults and with patients who have concurrent health and mental health problems.

This treatment manual is intended for health-care practitioners (psychologists, physicians, and nurses) and trainees who wish to develop competence in the assessment and treatment of insomnia. The goal is to reach health-care providers with a program that can be administered effectively in various clinical settings (e.g., outpatient clinics, primary care, and sleep disorders clinics). Special features were incorporated to make this book user-friendly and to ensure that it is utilized successfully as a therapy manual even by non-specialists. For example, clinical vignettes and summary boxes are inserted throughout to illustrate important conceptual and therapy features. In addition, key materials such as assessment scales, outlines of therapy sessions, and patient handouts and worksheets are available in the Appendixes and on an accompanying disk so they can be reproduced as needed.

We are very grateful to several individuals and organizations for their assistance in preparing this handbook. First, we are thankful to the numerous students, fellows, and trainees who have contributed to the development and validation of the materials presented in this book; their questions and ideas are always a source of challenge and stimulation for moving our field forward. We are also grateful to several funding organizations, including the Canadian Institute for Health Research, the Chief Scientist Office of the Scottish Executive Health Department, and the National Institute of Mental Health, for their financial support of our research programs over the last several years.

CHARLES M. MORIN
COLIN A. ESPIE

Contents

APPENDIXES

Insomnia
A Clinical Guide to Assessment and Treatment

Charles M. Morin
Université Laval
Quebec, Canada

and

Colin A. Espie
University of Glasgow
Glasgow, Scotland

Kluwer Academic / Plenum Publishers
New York Boston Dordrecht London Moscow

The Basics of Sleep

INTRODUCTION

This chapter provides an overview of some basic facts about normal sleep and the essential mechanisms and determinants regulating the sleep/wake cycle. The nature and organization of sleep are discussed first, followed by a summary of some biopsychosocial factors that may affect its quality and duration. Sleep needs are then examined, along with the consequences of sleep loss on daytime functioning, psychological well being, and physical health. As questions and concerns about the nature of sleep, sleep needs, and about the consequences of sleep loss are often brought up during insomnia treatment, it is important to establish basic knowledge about those issues early in the therapeutic process. This information should allow you and your patients to place insomnia in a common conceptual framework. It can also facilitate the patient's understanding, acceptance, and compliance with your treatment recommendations.

THE NATURE AND ORGANIZATION OF SLEEP

Sleep can be objectively studied by using polysomnography, a technique combining the measurement of brain activity (electroencephalography or EEG), eye movements (electro-occulography), and muscle tone (electromyography). Using this technique, two types of sleep can be distinguished: non-rapid-eye-movement (NREM) and rapid-eye-movement (REM) sleep, which are organized in a series of sleep cycles during the night. Different brain wave patterns detected during NREM sleep can be subdivided into four distinct sleep stages, simply labeled stages 1, 2, 3, and 4. From a state of drowsiness, the individual slips into stage 1, then progresses sequentially through the other stages of NREM sleep. Of short duration (about 5 minutes), stage 1 is a transitional phase between wakefulness and more definite sleep. During this light sleep, the arousal threshold is low and the brain wave signal is characterized by low-amplitude and high frequency waves. Progressively, the amplitude of the signal increases and its frequency decreases as the individual enters subsequent NREM stages. Stage 2 lasts 10 to 15 minutes and, for most people, corresponds to the phenomenological experience of falling asleep. Stages 3 and 4 are considered the deepest stages of sleep and together last between 20 to 40 minutes in the first sleep cycle. They are often referred to as "delta," or "slow-wave sleep" because of the presence of slow EEG waves of high amplitude called delta waves. After reaching stage 4, the EEG pattern reverses through stage 3, stage 2, and finally gives place to the first REM sleep episode (Carskadon & Dement, 2000).

In REM sleep, the EEG pattern is very similar to the one observed in stage 1. Brain waves of low-amplitude and high frequency are, however, accompanied by rapid movements of the eyes under the lids. The REM stage is often referred to as "paradoxical sleep" because it is characterized by a loss of core muscle tone while the activity in the brain and in the autonomic system are at a level similar to that seen during wakefulness. Apart from occasional muscle twitches, the body is essentially paralyzed in this stage. The most vivid dreams occur during REM sleep, even though non-narrative dream-like activity may also be recalled when subjects are woken up from the NREM stages. Even when dreams are not remembered, REM episodes and dream activity nonetheless occur during a normal night of sleep.

In healthy young adults who follow a regular sleep schedule, the proportion of time spent in REM sleep is about 25%, while the remaining 75% is spent in NREM sleep. NREM Stage 1 represents about 5%, Stage 2 another 50%, and Stages 3–4 about 20%. As shown in Figure 1.1, the distribution of sleep stages follows a highly structured and well-organized cyclic pattern, with slow-wave sleep occurring mainly in the first third of the night and REM sleep becoming more prominent and more intense in the latter part of the night and early morning hours. As we will see in the next section, the proportion of time spent in each stage of sleep, as well as sleep quality and quantity, can be altered by several factors, most notably, advancing age.

BIOPSYCHOSOCIAL DETERMINANTS OF SLEEP

Circadian and Homeostatic Factors

The propensity to sleep and the type of sleep experienced are highly dependent on circadian and homeostatic factors. Sleep is just one of many

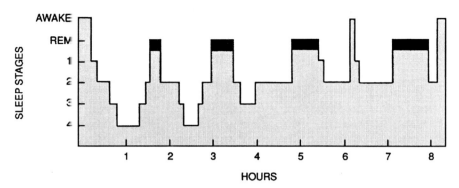

Figure 1.1. Sleep histogram. *Source*: C.M. Morin (1993). *Insomnia: Psychological Assessment and Management*, p. 17. New York: Guilford Press. Reprinted with permission.

biological functions (e.g., body temperature, melatonin and growth hormone secretion) that are regulated by circadian rhythms. A small brain structure located in the hypothalamus, serves as a biological clock to regulate this alternation between different states while interacting closely with time cues provided by the environment. The light-dark cycle is the most important of these cues. Social interactions, work schedules, and meal times are other extrinsic time cues that also contribute to regulating our sleep-wake cycles. Homeostatic factors can also impact significantly on sleep. For instance, the time to fall asleep is inversely related to the duration of the previous period of wakefulness. With prolonged sleep deprivation, there is an increasing drive to sleep. Upon recovery, there is a rebound effect producing a shorter sleep latency, increased total sleep time, and a larger proportion of slow-wave sleep. Following sleep loss, there is a preferential recovery of slow-wave sleep, followed by REM sleep (Billard, 1994).

Daily variations in core body temperature, which are also controlled by circadian factors, are closely tied to sleep-wake patterns (Czeisler & Khalsa, 2000). At its lowest point in the early hours of the day (e.g., 3:00 to 5:00 a.m.), body temperature starts to rise near the time of awakening and peaks in the evening. Alertness is at its maximum during the ascending slope of the body temperature curve. In contrast, sleepiness and sleep itself occur as temperature decreases. In the absence of time cues or any schedule constraint, individuals tend to choose a bedtime that is closely linked to a decrease in body temperature, while awakening occurs shortly after it begins to rise again. There is a slight drop in temperature in mid-afternoon, which can be associated with a temporary decline in alertness and a prime time for falling asleep.

These basic facts about homeostatic and circadian principles have important implications for understanding sleep problems as well as difficulties with staying awake. For night-shift workers, even those who sleep well during the day, it is often very difficult to stay alert around 3:00 or 4:00 a.m. because of decreased body temperature at that time. For the same reason, truck accidents are proportionally more frequent during early morning hours, despite less dense traffic during these hours. Conversely, body temperature tends to remain higher throughout the night in insomniacs, compared to good sleepers, explaining partly their difficulties sleeping. Some insomnia subtypes are linked to an abnormal circadian rhythm of body temperature. For example, one subgroup of sleep-onset insomniacs is characterized by a delayed sleep phase syndrome, a condition associated with a delay in the temperature drop at night (Morris, Lack, & Dawson, 1990). Conversely, older adults tend to become sleepy earlier in the evening than younger people, reflecting a natural phase advance in circadian rhythm with advancing age.

Age and Maturation

Age is probably the single most important variable determining the quality and duration of sleep (Carskadon & Dement, 2000). Figure 1.2 illustrates the main changes in sleep patterns with aging. Newborns need about 16 to 18 hours of sleep distributed in several episodes throughout the day and night. From early childhood to late adolescence, the sleep-wake cycle becomes progressively organized into a single nocturnal episode of about 9.5 hours of sleep. Then, total sleep time decreases gradually to level off in early adulthood at an average of 7 to 8.5 hours per night. Changes in the sleep architecture occur very gradually with the maturation process occurring throughout the life span.

The most important change is with REM sleep, which occupies more than 50% of total sleep time in newborns compared to 25% in young adults. There is also a decrease in the amount of stages 3–4 sleep and an increase in the number of awakenings. These changes become more noticeable in the forties. In later life, nocturnal sleep is diminished but, with daytime naps, total sleep time is often maintained at about 7 hours per 24-hour period. Nonetheless, sleep quality is diminished with aging, as there is a marked reduction of deep sleep and an increase of time spent in stages 1 and 2. Older adults experience more frequent and prolonged awakenings, which may explain the increased incidence of sleep complaints in this population. In addition, older adults tend to spend more time in bed, often in an attempt to meet their perceived sleep needs. Because a significant proportion of that time is actually spent awake, sleep becomes less efficient

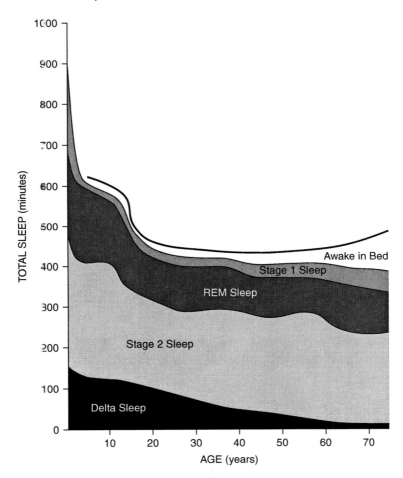

Figure 1.2 Changes in Sleep Patterns with Aging. *Source*: P.J. Hauri (1982). *The sleep disorders.* Kalamazoo, MI: Upjohn. Reprinted with permission.

with aging. As we will see later, an important component of behavioral treatment of insomnia in older adults consists of restricting the amount of time spent in bed in order to consolidate sleep over a shorter period of time.

Medical Conditions and Drugs

Sleep is vulnerable to medical illnesses. Disturbed sleep is often one of the first signs of an infection or a medical disorder. A variety of endocrine (e.g., hyperthyroidism), cardiovascular (e.g., congestive-heart failure), neurological (e.g., Parkinson's disease), and pulmonary diseases (e.g., chronic obstructive pulmonary disease) can disrupt sleep-wake functions. Sleep disturbances very frequently accompany medical conditions producing pain (e.g., arthritis, cancer, and chronic pain syndrome). Indeed, pain-inducing conditions, particularly fibromyalgia, have been associated with frequent intrusions of wakefulness into NREM sleep, a condition called alpha-delta sleep (Moldofsky, 1989).

Numerous prescribed and over-the-counter drugs can alter sleep patterns. Some medications prescribed for medical conditions may cause insomnia (e.g., bronchodilators, steroids) and others may produce sleepiness (e.g., antihistamines). Most psychotropic medications have a marked impact on sleep. Sedative-hypnotics have sleep promoting effects, but they also alter the underlying sleep architecture. For instance, benzodiazepines improve sleep continuity but they also increase stages 1 and 2 and decrease stages 3–4 sleep. Some antidepressant medications (e.g., amitryptiline, doxepin, trazodone) have sedating properties, while others (e.g., fluoxetine) have a more energizing effect and produce insomnia, and still others selectively suppress REM sleep. The time of administration of these pharmacological agents, as well as the duration of use, is often critical in determining how they will affect sleep. Your patients should consult their physicians and pharmacists to verify if the medications or products they use is likely to interfere with sleep.

Psychosocial Factors

Sleep is very sensitive to stress and emotional distress. Major life events such as a divorce or the death of a loved one, and more minor but daily stressors, like interpersonal difficulties or pressure at work, can affect sleep patterns by heightening arousal before falling asleep and during nocturnal awakenings (Morin, Rodrigue, & Ivers, 2003). Although sleep usually returns to normal once the acute stressful situation has resolved, sleep disturbances may become chronic due to a variety of perpetuating factors such as maladaptive habits or dysfunctional cognitions about sleep. There is also a clear association between sleep disturbances and psychopathology. Sleep disturbance is a symptom found in a variety of psychiatric disorders, most notably anxiety and depression, and the incidence of psychopathology is higher among individuals suffering from insomnia than in good sleepers (Ford & Kamerow, 1989). Although there is a definite link between psychological symptoms and sleep disturbances, it is often difficult to determine which is the cause and which is the consequence. We will return to this topic when we discuss differential diagnosis in the next chapter.

Lifestyle and Environmental Factors

Several lifestyle factors have noticeable repercussions on sleep patterns including diet, exercise, sleep schedules, and environmental conditions. For example, social drugs such as caffeine, nicotine, and alcohol can alter sleep when ingested too close to bedtime. The ingestion of heavy meals late in the evening can also disrupt sleep. Physical exercise can either promote or interfere with sleep, depending on its timing, intensity, and regularity, as well as the physical fitness of an individual. Exercising too close to bedtime will interfere with sleep, whereas a moderate amount of regular physical activity, scheduled late in the afternoon or early in the evening, may promote deep sleep. Daytime naps, particularly late in the day, will delay sleep onset for the following night. Long naps may produce deep sleep, which will be proportionally reduced during the next sleep episode. Environmental factors such as noise, temperature, light, and sleeping conditions (e.g., mattress quality) can also impact on sleep. Noise from traffic or from a snoring bed partner can lead to more disrupted sleep. A room temperature that is too hot or too cold will almost inevitably disrupt sleep. Chapter 4 outlines basic "sleep hygiene" recommendations that you should incorporate in the overall treatment plan in order to minimize the detrimental impact of lifestyle and environmental factors on sleep.

SLEEP NEEDS

The Functions of Sleep

Although several hypotheses have been proposed to explain the functions of sleep (see Horne, 1988), there is still no clear answer to the question "Why do we sleep?" Adaptive theories suggest that sleep has evolved as a protective mechanism to keep the organism out of danger during periods of inactivity. Proponents of a recuperative theory postulate that sleep serves a "maintenance" role through which the integrity of organic tissues and of psychic functions is restored. Still, other theories have suggested a role of sleep in processes such as energy conservation, regulation of body temperature, and immune functions. No single theory can account for the diversity and complexity of the processes that occur during sleep. Evidence from sleep deprivation studies suggests that NREM sleep, particularly Stages 3–4 sleep, is involved in restoration of physical energy, while REM sleep, aside from its presumed role in the resolution of emotional conflicts, has an important function in the consolidation of newly acquired memories. Whatever its exact role, sleep is as necessary as food and water. Indeed animals totally deprived of sleep during a prolonged period eventually die, suggesting that sleep serves a vital function in humans and animals.

Evaluating Individual Sleep Needs

A question that often arise in therapy is: How much sleep do I need? In addition to the effects of age and maturation previously described, sleep needs can be temporarily altered by other conditions such emergencies, work loads, pregnancy, travel, or medical illness. In general though, the average adult without insomnia complaint sleeps about 7–8 hours a night. There are, however, individual differences in sleep needs. Some people function well with as little as 4 or 5 hours of sleep while others need up to 9 or 10 hours to feel alert and energetic during the day. These patterns are usually quite stable throughout adulthood suggesting that individual sleep needs are probably determined genetically. How much sleep a given individual requires can be determined by varying sleep duration and testing how much time is needed in order to feel refreshed in the morning and alert throughout the next day. You will be able to actually test your patient's sleep needs when it is time to implement the sleep scheduling procedures (see Chapter 5).

Adequately fulfilling individual sleep needs has become more difficult in the last few decades. Indeed, while most activities were usually brought to a halt by nightfall before industrialization took place, today's society works on a different pace. Shops and factories are open day in and day out, and people often take on several jobs at a time, or combine work with familial responsibilities. Whereas the average sleep time was between 7 and 8.5 hours a night in the 1960's, today more than 50% of the population reports sleeping less than 7 hours. Making up for this slight sleep deprivation by napping or extending the sleep periods on weekends is not uncommon, but it is likely that many people live with a chronic sleep debt, i.e., with less sleep than they need.

THE CONSEQUENCES OF SLEEP DEPRIVATION

Insomnia patients often express concerns as to the possible detrimental effects of chronic sleep loss on their health, performance at work, and quality of life. It is important to make a clear distinction between the effects of persistent insomnia and the consequences of sleep deprivation. We begin this section with the effects of sleep deprivation and conclude with a brief discussion of the impact of insomnia. The effects of sleep deprivation depend on whether the sleep loss is total or partial, whether it is acute or chronic, and whether it is imposed by an emergency situation or caused by an underlying medical or psychiatric disorder.

Total Sleep Deprivation

Several studies have examined the effects of experimental sleep deprivation on physiological (e.g., sleepiness), psychological (e.g., mood, personality), and cognitive functioning (e.g., memory, reaction time, vigilance) (See Bonnet, 2000). The most prominent effect of total sleep deprivation is an increased feeling of sleepiness and desire for sleep. After one or two nights without sleep, most individuals show micro-sleep episodes intruding into wakefulness, which produce lapses of attention. Cognitive impairments are found mainly on tasks requiring sustained attention and rapid reaction time. Skills and processes involved in safe and vigilant driving are particularly sensitive to sleep deprivation, posing serious safety hazards. Executive functions such as judgement, creativity, and mental flexibility are also altered after prolonged sleep loss. Changes in mood have been noted after at least one night of total sleep deprivation. Individuals tend to be more irritable, and show less motivation, interest and initiative. Surprisingly, acute sleep deprivation has been found to have a transient antidepressant effect in persons with major depression; this effect is very short-lived as mood returns to baseline after the very first sleep episode. The few reports of personality changes or psychotic-like behaviors after prolonged sleep loss have been related to special contexts such as combat situations.

Partial Sleep Deprivation

Although total sleep deprivation for more than one night is relatively rare, partial sleep loss is far more common. Individuals with chronic pain syndromes or sleep apnea often show a fragmentation of their sleep and frequent awakenings, which are followed by severe daytime sleepiness. Likewise, many individuals who function on less sleep than they need, because of occupational or family obligations, may accumulate a chronic sleep debt. The consequences of prolonged sleep deprivation, even partial, can be very serious with regard to cognitive performance, quality of life, and public health safety. For example, in situations where sustained attention is needed, while driving or while operating heavy industrial machinery, partially sleep deprived individuals may put themselves and others at great risk. Several major accidents (e.g., Exxon Valdez, Chernobyl nuclear plant) have been linked to fatigue and sleep deprivation (Dinges, 1995).

Insomnia, Sleep Loss, and Daytime Functioning

In persistent primary insomnia, the actual sleep loss is usually less pronounced than what would be expected based on the patient's subjective complaint, and also less than what is observed in other sleep disorders such as sleep apnea or narcolepsy. While fatigue is almost always present in insomnia, excessive daytime sleepiness, the key marker of insufficient sleep, is not. In fact, insomnia patients typically report being unable to sleep, not only at night, but also when trying to nap during the day. The reason may be that they tend to remain in a chronic state of hyperarousal or hypervigilance. In addition, insomnia patients often perceive their performance as sub-optimal and they report decrements in their cognitive performance (e.g., memory, attention, concentration). However, these subjective complaints are not always entirely corroborated by objective findings (Vignola, Lamoureux, Bastien, Morin, 2000). Indeed, there is only limited evidence that, under experimental conditions, insomnia patients exhibit significant performance decrements on tests of memory, executive functions, or even attention and concentration (Riedel & Lichstein, 2000). The generalizability of those findings from laboratory-experiments to real-life situations can be questioned however. Also, current neuropsychological measures may not be sensitive enough to detect subtle deficits in insomnia.

Impact of Insomnia on Psychological Well-Being

Despite the absence of significant daytime sleepiness and only limited evidence of cognitive impairments in insomnia patients, chronic sleep disturbances in insomnia may nevertheless have a detrimental impact on psychological well-being and quality of life (Espie, 1991). Indeed, insomnia is almost always associated with fatigue and mood disturbances such as irritability and dysphoria. The unpredictable and uncontrollable nature of sleep can lead some individuals to present with irritability, tension, helplessness or even depressed mood. Longitudinal studies have suggested that untreated persistent insomnia may even be a risk factor for developing major depression (e.g., Ford & Kamerow, 1989). Sleep loss in insomnia can thereby cause considerable distress, impact on professional and social functioning, and decrease quality of life. In turn, these emotional disturbances may contribute to insomnia patient's feelings of fatigue, decreased performance, and mood alterations.

Impact of Insomnia on Physical Health

Insomnia patients will often come into therapy with great concerns about the impact of sleeplessness on their physical health. Somatic complaints most frequently reported by individuals with insomnia include gastrointestinal problems, respiratory problems, as well as headaches and non-specific aches and pain. Although there is a strong association between sleep and health complaints (Katz & McHorney, 1988), no clear causal relationship has been established yet. Some patients may fear that persistent insomnia will eventually result in a major medical illness such as a stroke or even cancer. In humans, there is little evidence that sleep loss, even for several days, produces any permanent or severe physical dysfunction. Some studies have suggested that chronic sleep deprivation may diminish immune function, yet no clear causal relationship has emerged with clinical insomnia (Savard et al., 2003). The psychological distress associated with sleep loss, rather than the sleep loss per se, may contribute to lowering immune function. Sleep duration has been linked to longevity, either short (4 hours or less) or long (10 hours or more) sleep durations being correlated with a higher mortality rate, but insomnia itself has not been associated with longevity.

In summary, this chapter has outlined some basic facts about normal sleep and its determinants, and about sleep needs and the consequences of sleep deprivation. Important distinctions were made between the consequences of sleep deprivation and those associated with insomnia. Establishing these basic facts early on in therapy may help diminish your patients' anxiety and, in turn, create a more favorable climate for initiating therapy and promoting compliance with the treatment procedures. For some patients, it will be necessary to rely on a systematic cognitive restructuring approach to modify some erroneous beliefs. It will be important, however, to prepare adequately your patients and find the appropriate timing for confronting some of those beliefs your patients may have about sleep and the impact of sleep loss and insomnia on daytime functioning. We will return to this in chapter 6 when addressing cognitive therapy.

Clinical Features of Insomnia

INTRODUCTION

This chapter describes the main features of insomnia, including the nature of the presenting complaints, associated clinical and psychological symptomatology, and polysomnographic and neuropsychological findings. Criteria to evaluate the severity and clinical significance of insomnia are also described. This background information is intended to provide you as a clinician with the essential features of insomnia in order to facilitate the initial assessment of your patients and to evaluate treatment outcome.

CLINICAL PRESENTATION

Vignette 1. Donna is a 34-years-old single female and high school teacher who presents to the sleep clinic with a chief complaint of difficulties falling asleep. She goes to bed at 10:30 p.m. but rarely falls asleep before 1:00 a.m. Once asleep, she can stay asleep until the next morning. She complains of mental fatigue and feels that her insomnia greatly impairs her abilities to concentrate and to teach effectively during the day. She displays significant sleep anticipatory anxiety and feels her sleep is totally unpredictable. She states that it is always the same film of anxious thoughts, mixed with mundane events, that keeps unrolling through her mind and prevents her from falling asleep. She's tried staying focused on her breathing or just making her mind blank, but nothing seems to work to get rid of those intrusive thoughts. Although sleep was disturbed only occasionally at first, it is now a more frequent problem and it seems to get worst all the time.

Vignette 2. Steve, a 43-years-old executive, doesn't have any trouble falling asleep. He is so exhausted when he goes to bed around 11:30 that he usually falls asleep in 5 minutes. His problem is that he doesn't stay asleep. He wakes up two or three times a night, for no apparent reason, and has difficulties getting back to sleep. Upon awakening, he thinks about unfinished business at the office or what is on the agenda for the next day. Eventually, he returns to sleep, only to wake up again an hour or so later. He has come to expect that if he wakes up, he will be awake for at least 30–45 minutes. Although he didn't think much of this as a problem initially, this is taking its toll in the long run and is affecting both his performance at work and his energy and interest in participating in social and family activities. He is very dissatisfied with the interrupted quality of his sleep and is concerned about the consequences of this sleep problem on his daytime functioning and quality of life. In addition to fatigue and reduced energy, he is beginning to show other depressive symptoms.

Vignette 3. Unlike Donna and Steve, Henry, a 68-years-old retired and widower can fall asleep easily and stay asleep for about 5 or 6 hours. His main problem is that he wakes up too early in the morning, typically at 4:00 or 5:00, and can't get back to sleep at all. He gets up to go to the bathroom and quickly returns to bed, hoping he might be able to go back to sleep. It rarely works. So, he lays in bed awake and starts reminiscing about his life in general, the unexpected death of his wife two years ago, problems with his health, etc. Even after the clock goes off, he stays in bed until at least 7:00 a.m. Henry is concerned about this problem and feels he needs more sleep to function and enjoy life.

Vignette 4. Mary is a 53-year-old women who claims she has always been a poor sleeper. Since the onset of her menopause two-years ago, her sleep has become even more disrupted. Although she does not report a clear problem in falling or staying asleep, she feels that her sleep is light and of unrefreshing quality. She keeps a fairly regular sleep schedule, going to bed at 11:00 p.m. and arising at 6:30 a.m., but does not have the impression of getting into a solid, sound sleep. She reports to sleep at most 3–4 hours per night; she feels that she does not disconnect from her environment and that her brain continues to work throughout the night. A sleep study reveals only mild to moderate sleep continuity impairments, with a latency to persistent sleep of 25 minutes and an additional 45 minutes of wakefulness after sleep onset, for an overall sleep efficiency of 83%. Total sleep time is near 6 hours. Except for an increased of Stage 1 sleep (10%), and some evidence of alpha intrusion into NREM sleep, the overall proportions of time spent in the different sleep stages are within normal limits.

As these four clinical vignettes illustrate, insomnia entails a spectrum of complaints reflecting dissatisfaction with the quality, duration, or continuity of sleep. The presenting complaint may involve problems with falling asleep initially at bedtime (as with Donna), waking up in the middle of the night and having difficulty going back to sleep (Steve), or waking up too early in the morning with an inability to return to sleep (Henry). Sleep may also be described as light, poor, and non-restorative (Mary). These difficulties can be present either alone or in combination. In fact, mixed sleep onset and maintenance insomnia is probably more common than either type of difficulties alone. In addition, there can be extensive night-to-night variability in sleep patterns and the type of sleep difficulties may also change over the course of the disorder.

Subjective insomnia complaints are not always entirely corroborated by objective (polysomnographic) measures of sleep, as illustrated by our fourth vignette above (Mary). Such discrepancies illustrate that alteration in the perception of sleep is an important feature of insomnia. Supported or not by objective polysomnographic findings, insomnia is usually accompanied by reports of daytime fatigue, mixed anxiety and depressive features or other mood disturbances (e.g., irritability), and impairments of functioning during the day. It is often the concerns about those daytime impairments or about the impact of sleep disturbances on one's health, rather than insomnia per se, that prompt patients to seek treatment. On the other hand, it is important to note that some people with insomnia symptoms (i.e., delayed sleep onset or nocturnal awakenings) are not concerned about such symptoms nor do they perceive that it interferes with their functioning. These individuals are probably never seen in the clinic. Also, insomnia may not always present as a specific, or as the only, complaint. It is often embedded with another chronic problem underlying or sitting alongside other difficulties.

In summary, then, the main diagnostic criteria for insomnia (Table 2.1) involve a *subjective* complaint of difficulties initiating and/or maintaining sleep, or nonrestorative sleep, associated with marked distress and/or significant impairments of social or occupational functioning (APA, 1994; ASDA, 1997).

Table 2.1. Diagnostic Criteria for Primary Insomnia

- A subjective complaint of difficulties initiating or maintaining sleep, or nonrestorative sleep.
- Duration of insomnia is longer than 1 month.
- The sleep disturbance (or associated daytime fatigue) causes marked distress or impairment in social, occupational or other important areas of functioning.
- The sleep disturbance does not occur exclusively in the context of another mental or sleep disorder and is not the direct physiologic effect of a substance or a general medical condition.

DEFINITION

In addition to standard diagnostic criteria, several markers can be used to define insomnia more operationally and to evaluate its clinical significance (Table 2.2). These indicators include the severity, frequency, and duration of sleep difficulties and their associated daytime consequences. For example, the amount of time required to fall asleep and the duration of awakenings are useful markers of insomnia severity. Sleep-onset insomnia and sleep-maintenance insomnia are respectively defined by a latency to sleep onset and/or time awake after sleep onset greater than 30 minutes, with a corresponding sleep efficiency (ratio of time asleep over time spent in bed multiplied by 100) lower than 85 percent. Likewise, early morning awakening can be defined by an awakening occurring earlier (more than 30 minutes) than desired, with an inability to go back to sleep, and before total sleep time reaches 6.5 hours. Because of individual differences in sleep needs, total sleep time is not a good index to define insomnia when considered alone. As we have discussed before, some people may function well with as little as 5–6 hours of sleep and would not necessarily complain of insomnia, while others needing 9–10 hours may still complain of inadequate sleep. These criteria, while arbitrary, are useful to operationalize a subjective complaint of insomnia.

It is also important to consider the frequency and duration of sleep difficulties to quantify insomnia severity. You must distinguish the occasional insomnia that everyone experiences at one time or another in life from the more frequent or persistent insomnia. The usual cut-off point is three nights or more per week with difficulties initiating and/or maintaining sleep; however, there may be extensive variability in sleep patterns, such that sleep may be disrupted 4–5 nights on a given week, followed by a good week with only 1–2 nights of insomnia. A distinction is also made between situational/acute insomnia, a condition lasting a few days and often associated with life events or jet lag, short-term/subacute insomnia (lasting between one and four weeks), and persistent insomnia,

Table 2.2. Criteria for Defining Insomnia

- *Severity of sleep disturbances*: Sleep latency or time awake after sleep onset greater than 30 min; or, last awakening occurring more than 30 min before desired time and before total sleep time reaches 6.5 hours; sleep efficiency is lower than 85%. May not be corroborated by PSG findings.
- *Frequency*: Sleep difficulties present three or more nights per week.
- *Duration*: Insomnia present for more than 1 (DSM-IV) or 6 months (ICSD).
- *Daytime impairments/marked distress*: Score of 2 or 3 on Insomnia Severity Index scale (items 5 and 7).

---

lasting more than one month. It is also necessary to consider the impact of insomnia on a person's life to judge its clinical significance as some people do experience sleep disturbances without any significant negative consequences. The most frequent complaints associated with insomnia, as stated earlier, involve fatigue, difficulties with attention and concentration, memory problems, and mood disturbances. Finally, the degree of distress is important to evaluate as some otherwise good sleepers can experience occasional sleep disturbances without being distressed about it.

CONCOMITANT LABORATORY FINDINGS AND CLINICAL FEATURES

The diagnosis of insomnia is predominantly based on the patient's subjective complaints. Although polysomnography is not readily available to non-sleep clinicians, laboratory findings can be very informative to document the extent to which objective evidence corroborate the subjective complaint of nighttime sleep disturbances.

Polysomnographic (PSG) Findings

It is well recognized that there is a natural tendency for both poor and good sleepers to overestimate the amount of time spent awake and to underestimate the amount of time spent asleep at night. The extent of those discrepancies between subjective and objective findings seem to follow a continuum (Edinger & Fins, 1995). They are probably present to some extent in all forms and subtypes of insomnia, with the most extreme cases diagnosed with a condition called "sleep-state misperception" (i.e., subjective insomnia without any PSG evidence of disrupted sleep). Aside from this subgroup of individuals with pure sleep-state misperception, PSG findings in subjectively-defined insomniacs generally reveal more impairments of sleep continuity parameters (i.e., longer sleep latencies, more time awake after sleep onset, lower sleep efficiency) and reduced total sleep time compared to subjectively-defined good sleepers. Also, insomniacs tend to spend more time in stage 1 sleep, less time in stages 3–4 sleep, and display more frequent stage shifts through the night. Investigations of the microstructure of sleep reveal that fast EEG (beta) activity is increased in primary insomnia relative to good sleepers, both around the sleep onset period and during NREM sleep (Merica, Blois & Gaillard, 1998; Perlis, Smith, Andrews, Orff & Giles, 2001). These latter findings are consistent with psychological data showing that insomniacs are hypervigilant and ruminative at sleep onset and/or during sleep and with the presumed role of attentional processes and information processing factors (Perlis et al., 2001).

Interestingly, sleep disturbances recorded in primary insomniacs are similar to those observed in patients with generalized anxiety disorders or some affective disorders such as dysthymia (Hauri & Fisher, 1986; Reynolds et al., 1984), suggesting a common underlying thread to these conditions. In addition, there is a significant overlap in the distribution of PSG sleep findings of subjectively-defined insomniacs and good sleepers such that some insomniacs may show better objective sleep than good sleepers and some good sleepers more sleep impairments than insomniacs. Once again, this paradox highlight the importance of the subjective complaint to make an insomnia diagnosis.

Fatigue and Sleepiness

The complaint of fatigue is almost always associated with insomnia. Although patients may complain of excessive daytime sleepiness, a more in depth investigation usually reveals that insomniacs experience mental and physical fatigue rather than true physiological sleepiness. Findings from the Multiple Sleep Latency Test of primary insomniacs are often comparable to those of good sleepers (Stepanski, Zorich, Roehrs, Young & Roth, 1988; see Chapter 3 for more information on the MSLT). Excessive daytime sleepiness is more common among patients with insomnia secondary to another medical (e.g., pain) or sleep disorders (e.g., periodic limb movements, sleep-related breathing disorders) compared to those with primary insomnia. The latter group experiences trouble sleeping at night, in part because of a chronic hyperarousal state, which also interferes with their ability to nap during the day.

Psychological Profile

The large majority of individuals seen in treatment for insomnia present at least some psychological symptoms of anxiety and/or depression (Edinger et al., 2000; Espie, 1991; Morin, 1993). The most classic psychological feature involves a form of sleep anticipatory anxiety (usually about not being able to sleep), which often leads to a conditioned arousal at bedtime. Excessive worrying about lack of sleep and its potential consequences is another common feature. There is also a form of learned helplessness or dysphoria that may develop when insomnia is persistent. This latter feature may become more apparent when an individual with persistent sleep difficulties perceives that, regardless of what he does, sleep remains unpredictable and uncontrollable. There may also be some more enduring traits such as ruminative, worry-prone, or even dysthymic-like personality traits. Despite the high prevalence of such psychological features, these symptoms do not always exceed diagnostic threshold for anxiety or depressive disorders. In fact, it is not always easy for the clinician to determine the extent to which such features are causes or consequences of insomnia. We will discuss those features in greater details when addressing the differential diagnosis of insomnia.

Neuropsychological Findings

Most individuals seen in consultation for insomnia report impairments of their mental abilities involving attention/concentration, memory, and executive functions. However, objective evaluations of the daytime performance of insomnia research participants usually reveal only mild and fairly selective deficits (Riedel & Lichstein, 2000). It is unclear whether clinical patients present more objective daytime deficits than those solicited for research studies. Nonetheless, insomniacs tend to have lower expectations and to rate their performance as significantly impaired relative to their own standards (i.e., what they should be able to do) and as more impaired than that of normal controls. Those discrepancies between subjective and objective performance are similar to those observed between subjective and objective measures of sleep. As such, they may reflect a generalized faulty appraisal of sleep and daytime functioning among individuals with insomnia complaints (Vignola et al., 2000). Another paradoxical finding is that performance impairments on neuropsychological testing are more strongly associated with subjective (as measured by daily sleep diaries) than with objective (as measured by PSG) sleep disturbances. Such findings illustrate the complexity of insomnia and may explain why some individuals with insomnia symptoms do not complain about it, whereas others are dissatisfied with their sleep in the absence of significant sleep disturbances. Collectively, these findings suggest that the subjective appraisal/perception of sleep and daytime functioning are partly modulated by psychological and cognitive factors which, in turn, are important determinants of insomnia complaints.

COURSE AND PROGNOSIS

Insomnia can be situational, recurrent, or persistent. The type of insomnia may also change over time, with sleep onset difficulties being more typical of the first episodes of insomnia and sleep maintenance difficulties becoming more common in the later phase of the disorder. The first episode of insomnia may occur at any age, with either a sudden or insidious onset, but individuals with primary insomnia report most frequently that they first experienced sleep difficulties during their 20's or early 30's (Morin, 1993). That first episode of insomnia is often associated with a stressful life event (e.g., school exam, new job, and birth of a child) (Bastien, Vallières, & Morin, in press). Subsequently, sleep may have normalized for a few weeks, months, or even years but, eventually, sleep disturbances have returned more frequently or for longer periods.

For the majority of individuals, sleep difficulties are transient in nature, lasting a few days, and resolving themselves once the initial precipitating event has subsided. For some people, however, perhaps those with a higher predisposition to insomnia, sleep disturbance may persist over time even after the initial cause has disappeared. Insomnia may follow an intermittent course, with repeated brief episodes of sleep difficulties following a close association with the occurrence of stressful events or, it may become a chronic problem (Vollrath, Wicki, & Angst, 1989). Even in persistent insomnia, there is often extensive night-to-night variability in sleep, with an occasional good night's sleep intertwined with several nights of disrupted sleep. This unpredictability of sleep can be very distressing and it may eventually induce a sense of learned helplessness.

The long-term prognosis of untreated insomnia is not well documented. However, there is some evidence suggesting that insomnia is often a recurrent problem and, when left untreated, it increases the risks for major depression (Ford & Kamerow, 1989). Even with treatment, some patients will continue to experience intermittent sleep difficulties. For this reason, it is particularly important to teach patients appropriate behavioral and coping skills to manage those residual episodes of insomnia and reduce the risk of chronicity and morbidity associated with insomnia.

INSOMNIA AS A SYMPTOM OR A SYNDROME

Insomnia may present as an isolated symptom, as a cluster of symptoms that remain sub-clinical, or it may exceed diagnostic threshold and meet criteria for a full clinical syndrome. In the first scenario, there may be occasional difficulties falling or staying asleep (e.g., on Sunday night or before an important deadline), which may or may not be perceived as problematic. When sleep difficulties are present once or twice a week and are associated with daytime impairments, they may produce more distress but are still considered sub-clinical. When they exceed diagnostic threshold, insomnia is considered a full clinical syndrome, which may be primary or secondary in nature.

The two main nosological classifications of sleep disorders (ICSD and DSM-IV) make an essential distinction between primary and secondary insomnia. In secondary insomnia, the sleep disturbance is etiologically linked to an underlying condition, including psychiatric, medical, substance abuse, and other sleep disorders. As such, it is usually seen as a symptom or a cluster of symptoms that are predominantly caused by the underlying condition. In primary insomnia, the sleep disturbance does not occur exclusively in the context of another medical, psychiatric, or substance abuse disorders; it may co-exist with these conditions but it is viewed as an independent disorder (Buysse et al., 1994). Individuals with primary insomnia may show anxiety and depressive symptomatology, but such clinical findings are not severe enough to reach diagnostic threshold for an anxiety or affective disorder. They are viewed as consequence or co-existing symptoms rather than causes of insomnia. A rough estimate is that approximately one third of individuals with insomnia presents another psychopathology, one third presents significant psychological symptoms without exceeding diagnostic threshold, and about one third do not show significant psychological symptoms. Because of the high rate of comorbidity between sleep disturbances and psychopathology, the determination of whether insomnia is cause or consequence is not always easy to make to reach an accurate differential diagnosis.

Differential Diagnosis between Primary and Secondary Insomnia

The diagnosis of insomnia is often made by default, after all other possible contributing conditions have been ruled out. Because of the frequent co-existence of anxiety and depressive symptoms, it is sometimes difficult to make an accurate differential diagnosis between primary insomnia and insomnia secondary to anxiety and depressive disorders. As illustrated in Figure 2.1, those three conditions share several symptoms in common including sleep disturbances, fatigue and decreased energy, and concentration problems. As part of the clinical evaluation, it is essential to conduct a detailed analysis of other clinical symptoms in order to determine if insomnia is primary or secondary in nature. In primary insomnia, patients often report excessive worries, but such concerns are typically very focused on sleeplessness, whereas in generalized anxiety disorders (GAD), sleep is only one of several sources of preoccupations (e.g., health, family, finances, work). In GAD, worrying is also more excessive and less controllable than in insomnia alone. Fatigue and poor concentration may also be present in GAD, but those symptoms are usually the result of excessive worrying rather than poor sleep as in insomnia. In depression, the most prominent symptoms are sadness, decreased interest in activities or people a person used to enjoy, and several other somatic, cognitive and affective symptoms.

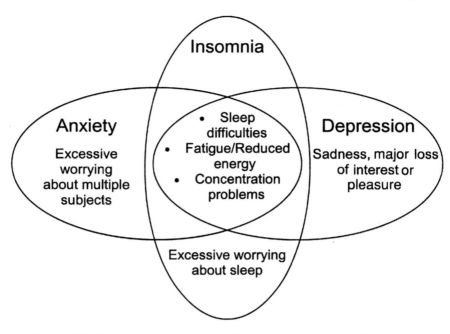

Figure 2.1. Overlapping symptoms of insomnia, anxiety, and depression.

In primary insomnia, the decreased level of activity is due to fatigue and poor sleep rather than to an intrinsic lack of interest as in depression. Another useful strategy to determine if insomnia is primary or secondary is to examine the temporal course of those conditions. Did the onset of insomnia precede the first depressive episode or the first appearance of other anxiety features? You should bear in mind, however, that it is often not reliable to conclude that insomnia is secondary to physical or mental health problems in a truly causal sense. In our view, the diagnostic criteria imply that insomnia is secondary when other problems predominate the overall clinical presentation. In many situations it might be more accurate to think of insomnia "associated with" another disorder because both presenting problems may merit attention.

Subtypes of Primary Insomnia

The DSM-IV recognizes only one form of primary insomnia, whereas the ICSD distinguishes among three different subtypes: psychophysiological insomnia, sleep-state misperception, and idiopathic insomnia. Psychophysiological insomnia, which is essentially the DSM-IV equivalent of primary insomnia, is the most classic form of insomnia. It is a type of conditioned or learned insomnia that is presumably derived from two sources. The first involves the conditioning of sleep-preventing habits in which repeated pairing of sleeplessness and situational (bed/bedroom), temporal (bedtime), or behavioral (bedtime ritual) stimuli normally associated with sleep leads to conditioned arousal that impairs sleep. The second involves somatized tension believed to result from the internalization of psychological conflicts and excessive worrying/apprehension about sleep, which are incompatible with sleep. The sleep of individuals with psychophysiological insomnia is very sensitive to minor irritants and daily stressors; it is also characterized by extensive night-to-night variability such that sleep is often unpredictable. Sometimes, their sleep is unexpectedly improved in a novel environment because the conditioned cues that keep them awake at home are not present in that environment. For example, while the sleep of otherwise good sleepers is more disrupted during their first night of recording in the sleep laboratory (i.e., first night effect), insomniacs may actually sleep better during their first night in the laboratory (i.e., the reverse first-night-effect).

Sleep-state misperception, also called subjective insomnia, is characterized by a genuine complaint of poor sleep that is not corroborated by objective findings. For example, a patient may perceive very little sleep (e.g., 1–2 hours per night) whereas PSG shows normal or near-normal sleep duration and quality. This sleep-state misperception condition is not the result of an underlying psychiatric disorder or of malingering. To some degree, all insomniacs tend to overestimate the time it takes them to fall asleep and to underestimate the time they actually sleep. In sleep-state misperception, however, the subjective complaint of poor sleep is clearly out of proportion with any objective finding. This phenomenon is probably due to several factors including the lack of sensitivity of EEG measures, the influence of cognitive (information processing) variables during the early stages of sleep or, it could also represents the far end of a continuum of individual differences in sleep perception. Interestingly, individuals with subjective insomnia report greater disruption of daily functioning than those with psychophysiological insomnia. Sleep-state misperception may be a prodromal phase for more objectively verifiable insomnia (Salin-Pascual, Roehrs, Merlotti, Zorick, & Roth, 1992). However, this condition is still poorly understood and some have suggested that it should not even be considered a separate diagnostic entity. The main problem with this diagnosis is that most clinicians do not have objective data to confirm or refute the patient's subjective complaint.

Idiopathic (childhood) insomnia is, by definition, of unknown origin. One of the most persistent forms of insomnia, it presents an insidious

Table 2.3. Clinical Features of Insomnia

- *Presenting complaints* (+++): Difficulties initiating or maintaining sleep; early morning awakening; light or unrefreshing sleep.
- *Associated features* (+++): Fatigue, impaired functioning, mixed anxious and depressive symptoms, dysphoria, anxiety-worry prone personality traits.
- *Polysomnographic findings* (++): Increased sleep latency and/or time awake after sleep onset, reduced sleep efficiency and total sleep time, increased Stages 1 and 2 and reduced Stages 3–4 sleep. Excessive sleepiness (+).
- *Neuropsychological findings*: Selected and mild impairments of attention/concentration (++), memory (+), and executive functions (+).

Note: Features that are present almost always (+++), sometimes (++), or rarely (+).

onset in childhood, unrelated to psychological trauma or medical disorders, and is very persistent throughout the adult life. It does not present the nightly variability observed with other forms of primary insomnia. Despite objective evidence of sleep disturbances and of daytime sequelae (e.g., memory, concentration and motivational difficulties), individuals with idiopathic insomnia may report less emotional distress than those with the psychophysiological subtype, perhaps due to coping mechanisms they have developed over their lifetime. On the other hand, this condition is sometimes associated with a dysthymic psychological profile. This form of insomnia has been hypothesized to stem from a mild defect of the basic neurological sleep/wake mechanisms; this hypothesis comes from the observations that patients with this condition often have a history of learning disabilities, attention-deficit hyperactivity, or similar conditions associated with minimal brain dysfunctions.

Despite some overlap among those three insomnia subtypes, this classification illustrates that insomnia does not always present as a single prototype. Rather, there are various insomnia profiles with significant variations regarding the presenting complaints, its associated features, and the temporal course of the condition. These different subtypes may also benefit from different treatments. For example, patients with sleep-state misperception may require interventions (e.g., cognitive therapy) that specifically seek to correct sleep misperceptions.

In summary, the essential features of insomnia include a *subjective* complaint of insomnia, present at least three nights per week and lasting a minimum of one month, and is associated with significant distress and/or impairments of daytime functioning. The subjective complaints of poor sleep and daytime impairments may or may not be corroborated by objective evidence from polysomnography and neuropsychological testing. In addition, insomnia is not always the presenting complaint in clinical practice; it can also be a non-specific complaint or an accessory complaint, which is embedded with another co-existing medical or psychiatric condition. Figure 2.1 provides some further useful information for you to bear in mind when you first see a new patient with insomnia.

DOES YOUR PATIENT SUFFER FROM INSOMNIA?

Before initiating therapy for insomnia, you must first acquire a global comprehension of your patient's condition by exploring its psychological, physiological, and behavioral dimensions. What are the nature and severity of your patient's complaint? How did the problem evolve with time? What are the potential causes of the sleep disturbance? Is there a medical or psychiatric underlying condition, or even a medication causing insomnia? What are the alleviating and exacerbating factors? Can another sleep pathology be producing the subjective complaint of insomnia? A careful assessment of insomnia complaints is needed to adequately guide patients along effective therapeutic avenues. The next chapter provides you with practical tools to successfully reach this goal.

Assessment and Differential Diagnosis of Insomnia

INTRODUCTION

In this chapter we will describe how to assess people with insomnia. Self-report, behavioral and physiological methods will be introduced, and issues of differential diagnosis from other sleep disorders will be explained. It is our intention that the text is practical, emphasizing how insomnia can be assessed and diagnosed in non-specialist healthcare settings where there is limited or no access to a sleep laboratory or sleep center. We would also draw your attention to the American Academy of Sleep Medicine review and practice parameters papers on the assessment of insomnia as a useful source of further information (Chesson et al., 2000; Sateiea, Doghramji, Hauri & Morin, 2000).

THE ASSESSMENT OF INSOMNIA

The Sleep History

The importance of "taking a history" is widely recognized in the clinical approach to any disorder, and insomnia is no exception. The history usually takes the form of an interview, enabling the clinician to obtain an overview of the problem. We have provided a format for a Sleep History interview in Table 3.1 (and Appendix A). This semi-structured approach guides you to use general, prompt questions to focus upon issues of interest, followed by more specific inquiry where required. It is during this interview that you will find out about the nature, developmental course

Table 3.1. Outline Plan for a Sleep History Assessment Comprising Content
Areas and Suggested Interview Questions

Content area	Prompt question	Supplementary questions
Presentation of the Sleep Complaint		
Pattern	Can you describe the pattern of your sleep on a typical night?	Time to fall asleep? Number and duration of wakenings? Time spent asleep? Nights per week like this?
Quality	How do you feel about the quality of your sleep?	Refreshing? Enjoyable? Restless?
Daytime effects	How does your night's sleep affect your day?	Tired? Sleepy? Poor concentration? Irritable? Particular times of day?
Development of the Sleep Complaint	Do you remember how this spell of poor sleep started?	Events and circumstances? Dates and times? Variation since then? Exacerbating factors? Alleviating factors? Degree of impact/intrusiveness?
Lifetime History of Sleep Complaints	Did you used to be a good sleeper?	Sleep in childhood? Sleep in adulthood? Nature of past episodes? Dates and times? Resolution of past episodes?
General Health Status and Medical History	Have you generally kept in good health?	Illnesses? Chronic problems? Dates and times? Recent changes in health?
Psychopathology and History of Psychological Functioning	Are you the kind of person who usually copes well?	Psychological problems? Anxiety or depression? Dates and times? Resourceful person? Personality type?
Issues of Differential Diagnosis		
Sleep-related breathing disorder (SBD)	Are you a heavy snorer?	Interrupted breathing in sleep? Excessively sleepy in the day?

Table 3.1. (*Cont.*)

Content area	Prompt question	Supplementary questions
Periodic limb movements in sleep (PLMS) and restless legs syndrome (RLS)	Do your legs sometimes twitch or can't keep still?	Excessively sleepy in the day? Trouble sitting still without moving the extremities?
Circadian rhythm sleep disorders	Do you feel you want to sleep at the wrong time?	Too early? Too late?
Parasomnias	Do you sometimes act a bit strangely during your sleep?	Behavioral description? Time during night?
Narcolepsy	Do you sometimes just fall asleep without warning?	Times and places? Collapses triggered by emotion? Poor sleep at night?
Current and Previous Treatments	Are you taking anything to help you sleep?	Now? In the past? Dates and times? What has worked? What have you tried yourself?

and impact of the sleep disorder. You will also be able to learn about current and previous interventions, including self-help strategies that the patient has used. Because assessment is conducted largely with a view to treatment, knowing what has been tried and for how long, and to what effect, is important (Morin, Gaulier, Barry & Kowatch, 1992). Experience may have an effect upon expectation of future therapy. Interviewing a spouse/partner may also be helpful, especially in relation to differential diagnosis, and we will say more about this later on.

If you are interested in looking at other broadly based assessment measures, there are several we can recommend. The Pittsburgh Sleep Quality Index (Buysse, Reynolds, Monk, Berman & Kupfer, 1989) is a widely used, and fairly brief questionnaire that patients can complete before they attend the clinic. It yields an index score of sleep quality and has a recognized threshold score (of > 5) that identifies significant sleep disturbance. Spielman and Anderson (1999) have developed a structured interview in which the interviewer rates symptoms in relation to International Classification of Sleep Disorders (ICSD) categories. The format ensures orderly consideration of psychological, social and physiological determinants of sleep disturbance. Finally, Morin (1993, pp. 195–198) has published an Insomnia Interview Schedule which is a practical tool for describing and recording the sleep complaint. It is particularly useful in the functional analysis of sleep behaviors, and also incorporates clinical diagnostic questions.

Table 3.2. Characteristics of the Sleep Diary

Features of sleep diaries	Comment
Practical usefulness	Sleep diaries are non-intrusive, inexpensive, adaptable to presenting need and acceptable to insomniacs to use. They are relatively simple to train, and are completed at home.
Clinical relevance	Sleep diaries permit prolonged measurement over weeks or months. This is helpful diagnostically to establish baselines and to assess change over time and at follow-up. They are relevant to all sleep disorders.
Validity and reliability	Sleep diaries enable quantification of the presenting sleep complaint, and qualitative information and measures of daytime effects can be incorporated. When compared with PSG data, diaries provide a reasonably reliable, relative index of sleep pattern.
Treatment relevance	Sleep diaries are essentially collaborative. The person with insomnia is engaged actively in the assessment process, and data are shared with the therapist. This is particularly useful in cognitive-behavioral treatment. They can be used to appraise treatment benefit.

The Sleep Diary

The Sleep Diary is invaluable in the appraisal of insomnia. Whereas the sleep history provides retrospective overview, the Sleep Diary yields night by night, self-report information on sleep pattern and quality that may be obtained over many weeks. The Sleep Diary has become the 'staple' of insomnia assessment and has stood the test of time. Sleep diaries have been in use since the early behavioral treatment studies and a number of commentaries on their advantages and disadvantages are available (Espie, 1991; Morin, 1993; Lichstein & Riedel, 1994). We have summarized the most important factors governing their use in Table 3.2, and examples of two Sleep Diary formats are presented in Figures 3.1 and 3.2.

In the diary, information on parameters such as time to bed, sleep-onset latency (SOL), frequency and total duration of wakenings (wake-time after sleep-onset; WASO), total sleep time (TST), waking and rising time is complemented by ratings of sleep quality. Although the diary in Figure 3.1 is more commonly used (reproduced also in Appendix B), the pictorial format (Figure 3.2) can be useful for diagnostic assessment; in the example given of a Delayed Sleep Phase Disorder (from Spielman & Anderson, 1999). We recommend that a Sleep Diary should be completed for about two weeks for the purposes of baseline assessment. We also suggest that some

	Day 1	Day 2	Day 3	Day 4	Day 5	Day 6	Day 7
MEASURING THE PATTERN OF YOUR SLEEP							
1. What time did you rise from bed this morning?							
2. At what time did you go to bed last night?							
3. How long did it take you to fall asleep (minutes)?							
4. How many times did you wake up during the night?							
5. How long were you awake *during* the night in total)?							
6. About how long did you sleep altogether (hours/mins)?							
7. How much alcohol did you take last night?							
8. How many sleeping pills did you take to help you sleep?							
MEASURING THE QUALITY OF YOUR SLEEP							
1. How well do you feel this morning? 0 1 2 3 4 not at all moderately very							
2. How enjoyable was your sleep last night? 0 1 2 3 4 not at all moderately very							

Name _____

Week Beginning _____

Figure 3.1. Example of a "standard" Sleep Diary incorporating information on sleep pattern and sleep quality. Numerical information is entered for each measure based upon the preceding night's sleep. Qualitative ratings can be personalized to suit the individual's own terminology regarding sleep

training is required to encourage patients in accurate reporting, whilst avoiding 'clockwatching' (Espie, 1991; pp. 75–77). Nevertheless, anxiety in using sleep diaries is usually transient, and most people find them easy to use and non-intrusive.

We believe that information from Sleep Diary assessment is valid primarily because it quantifies the actual complaint of insomnia. Retrospective, self-report measurement of any kind can, of course, be challenged,

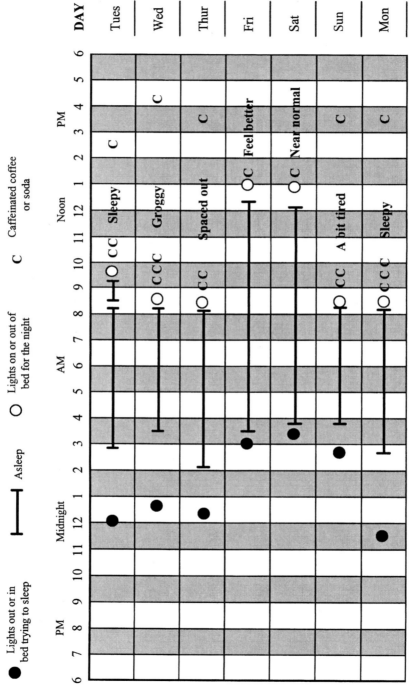

Figure 3.2. Example of a pictorial Sleep Diary where information is entered on the horizontal axis for each night's sleep. The case presented is indicative of Delayed Phase Disorder, illustrating one advantage of this format of Sleep Diary. *Source:* A.J. Spielman and M.W. Anderson (1999). *The clinical interview and treatment planning as a guide to understanding the nature of insomnia: The CCNY Interview for Insomnia* (p. 389). Copyright 1999 by Butterworth-Heinemann. Reprinted with permission.

and Sleep Diary assessment has been. However, research data indicate that diaries provide relatively reliable index measurements of sleep latency, wakefulness, sleep time and sleep efficiency (proportion of time in bed spent asleep). Although insomniacs generally over-report sleep disturbance, they tend to do so consistently. Besides, errors in estimation by insomniacs and normal sleepers can occur in both directions, and insomniacs usually have the more difficult self-report task (Espie, Lindsay & Espie, 1989; Edinger & Fins, 1995). Another important advantage is that diaries can be used continuously throughout intervention, so treatment-related change, and outcome, can be appraised against the patient's own baseline sleep disturbance.

Another useful measure is the Sleep Impairment Index (Morin, 1993), which has been validated and renamed the Insomnia Severity Index (ISI) (Bastien, Vallières, & Morin, 2001). Often we are interested not only in measuring the sleep problem itself, but also in appraising its severity and impact. The ISI is a 7-item scale on which the patient rates sleep difficulty in terms of its severity, degree of interference with daily functioning, noticeability of such impairment to others, level of distress, and overall satisfaction with sleep (Appendix C). The ISI can be completed at pre- and post-treatment as part of the evaluation of sleep improvement.

Informant Report

Interviewing an observer of sleep can be useful for two reasons. Firstly, to corroborate data from self-report; and secondly, to provide additional information which may assist diagnosis. In terms of the former, the partner may be able to confirm the frequency, severity and intrusiveness of a sleep disorder. However, partners are seldom able to provide accurate information on nighttime sleep; unless they too are insomniac! Other observers, such as nursing staff, have been used in hospital-based studies, however, such observation may be intrusive and precipitate sleep stage changes. Besides insomnia is seldom assessed in a hospital setting.

With respect to diagnosis, however, partner report can be crucial; for example, in sleep-related breathing disorder (SBD) where snoring, apneic episodes (respiratory pauses) and abrupt restoration of normal breathing may have been witnessed, or with periodic limb movement disorder (PLMD) where there are involuntary jerky movements. Partners may also provide important information on daytime functioning such as fatigue, sleepiness and mood, and on changes in symptoms over time.

Polysomnography

Polysomnography provides information on the sleeping/waking brain, and is the 'gold standard' for diagnostic assessment. Full polysomnography (PSG) comprises electroencephalography (EEG), electrooculography (EOG), chin and anterior tibialis electromyography (EMG), respiratory effort, airflow, oximetry and electrocardiography (ECG). Most assessments are laboratory-based and the first night of recording is usually discarded as comprising artifact due to the novelty of the procedure and environment. You might say the principles of stimulus control are recognized in practice. Because people sleep differently in a lab, and may have different attributions about their sleep, home PSG has been developed as a naturalistic alternative. The first portable PSG recordings were described in the 1970s but since then home recording has become simpler and more reliable. In insomnia research it is particularly important that the person sleeps in his/her own bed (Edinger et al., 1997).

PSG is critical to diagnosis in complex cases, and to monitoring the effects of interventions, such as nasal continuous airway pressure (nCPAP), where levels of oxygen saturation/desaturation, occurrences of apneas and frequent arousals from sleep have to be assessed before and during treatment. Expert reviews concur in recommending PSG where there are clinical grounds to suspect SBD, PLMD, persistent circadian disorders, precipitous arousals or violent behavior in sleep, and in other circumstances where the diagnosis remains uncertain. Routine PSG assessment, however, is not indicated for persistent insomnia (ASDA, 1995a; Reite, Buysse, Reynolds & Mendelson, 1995).

Actigraphy and Other Behavioral Devices

Body movement can be used to distinguish wakefulness from sleep, and conversely, the relative absence of movement is a reasonable correlate of sleep. Actigraphy was first introduced to sleep assessment more than 20 years ago, and contemporary devices are robust yet lightweight. They provide inexpensive, objective estimates of sleep over periods up to four weeks (Hauri & Wisbey, 1992; Sadeh, Hauri, Kripke & Lavie, 1995). The actigraph is attached to the non-dominant wrist and worn like a wristwatch. Interface units enable the downloading of data for graphing and sleep analysis. Continuous monitoring across 24-hour periods also permits analysis of daytime naps. Clearly, not all movement is wakefulness and not all absence of activity is sleep. Nevertheless, comparative studies with PSG have reported strong agreement for nocturnal sleep periods, and there is little evidence of a first night effect. Actigraphic evaluation is particularly

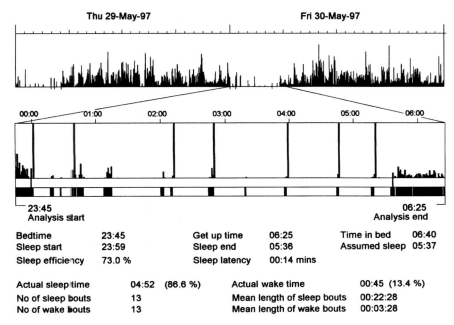

Figure 3.3. Twenty-four-hour wrist-actigraphic trace and sleep summary data from a 68-year-old woman with intermittent wakenings. Tall vertical lines represent perceived wakenings, entered by the subject by depressing an event marker button on the actigraph. (Actiwatch® Cambridge Neurotechnology Ltd., England)

useful for longitudinal study of circadian disorders of sleep (ASDA, 1995b; Chesson et al., 1997).

An example of an actigraphic tracing is reproduced in Figure 3.3. This 68-year-old woman was a 'light sleeper' and had intermittent arousals and unrestful, poor quality sleep. She did not experience problems in getting to sleep. Her Sleep Diary gave her bedtime as 11:45 p.m. and her rising time as 5:55 a.m. These parameters were used to set the 'window' for sleep analysis of actigraphic data. Inspection of the trace reveals several wakenings from sleep, 7 of which she identified by depressing an event marker on the actigraph. She had relatively short sleep (4 hours 52 min.) and scored 79% sleep efficiency. This example illustrates the usefulness of the actigraph in confirming self-report information.

We note also, that other behavioral responses may provide objective estimates of sleep pattern. Blood, Sack, Percy and Pen (1997) found that behavioral response monitoring (button-pressing contingent upon presentation of a low intensity tone) was more accurate in determining sleep latency than actigraphic assessment. Both procedures, however, were sensitive to the detection of sleep; and Lichstein and Johnson (1991) found a Sleep Assessment Device, which tape records verbal responses to preset, fixed interval tones, to be a useful and non-intrusive in the estimation of sleep.

Daytime Sleepiness

Persistent insomnia will not necessarily be associated with significant daytime sequelae, nevertheless, daytime sleepiness is medically significant as it may be a symptom of sleep apnea, narcolepsy, PLMD, circadian rhythm disorder, affective disorder, excessive drug or alcohol use, or idiopathic hypersomnolence. Experiences of 'tiredness' and 'sleepiness', therefore, should be differentiated. The latter can involve involuntary sleep or a likelihood of sleep occurring whilst engaged in routine activities. Fatigue by comparison comprises tiredness, lethargy, inattention and perhaps loss of motivation.

The Multiple Sleep Latency Test (MSLT) assesses, in a laboratory environment, the rapidity of sleep-onset during daytime nap opportunities, and has for long been the 'gold standard' measure of daytime sleepiness (Carskadon, Dement, Mitler, Roth & Westbrook, 1986). The MSLT, like PSG, is seldom required in the assessment of insomnia, but should be used when narcolepsy is suspected. Ratings of sleepiness, however, may be more widely used in routine practice. We recommend the Epworth Sleepiness Scale, an eight-item self-report measure commonly used in research and clinical practice with sleep apnea (ESS; Johns, 1991). This is reproduced in Appendix D. A high ESS score cannot be taken in isolation as evidence of SBD. Nevertheless, where there is a positive history and the partner has witnessed apneas, the probability of SBD is significantly increased. Cut-off points on the ESS of >11 for men and >9 for women have been taken as indicative of excessive daytime sleepiness (Whitney et al., 1998).

Predisposing, Precipitating and Perpetuating Factors

Before considering differential diagnosis, we want to introduce another useful framework within which insomnia can be assessed. Spielman & Glovinsky (1991) suggested a conceptualization comprising predisposing, precipitating and perpetuating components (Figure 3.4), and we feel that it may be helpful to consider each of these components as part of your clinical formulation.

Predisposing factors might include things like a familial association with light, disrupted sleep, or anxious over-concern with personal well being. Indeed, many insomniacs appear prone to introspection and worry.

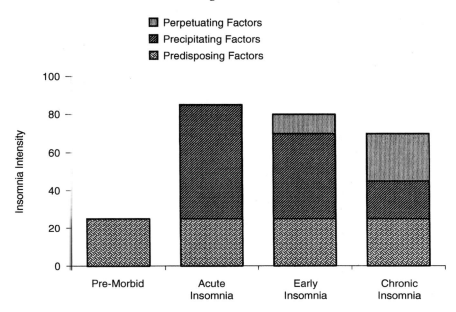

Figure 3.4. Predisposing, precipitating and perpetuating factors in insomnia. *Source*: A.J. Spielman and P.B. Glovinsky (1991). The varied nature of insomnia. In P.J. Hauri (Ed.) *Case studies of insomnia* (pp. 1–15). Copyright 1991 by Plenum Press. Reprinted with permission.

Research also suggests that elevated autonomic or metabolic rate may represent a vulnerability factor for insomnia. Nevertheless, predisposing factors alone would not normally produce insomnia. Transient sleep disorder seems a likely context within which to identify precipitating factors. Acute stress, conflict or environmental or occupational change may all be associated with sleep disturbance. However, if you take the view that acute insomnia will usually default to normal sleep after precipitating factors subside, because of the inherent 'plasticity' in the homeostatic processes which protect sleep (Espie, 2002), we need to consider perpetuating factors if we are to understand the presentation of persistent insomnia. Much of the psychological literature has focused on behavioral, cognitive and emotional factors, which may be associated with the persistence of insomnia, and these will be discussed in later chapters.

DIFFERENTIAL DIAGNOSIS OF INSOMNIA

Our view is that the effective sleep clinician works as a scientist-practitioner, using information to create and test hypotheses concerning

Table 3.3. Simplified Classification of Sleep Disorders to Aid Differential
Diagnosis of Insomnia

Sleep disorder	Summary description of disorder
Insomnia	Difficulty in initiating and/or maintaining sleep occurring 3 or more nights per week and persisting for at least 6 months. Possible daytime mood and performance effects.
Normal aging	Developmentally normal changes in sleep and wakefulness.
Sleep-Related Breathing Disorder (SBD)	Cessation of breathing (apnea), loud snoring, choking/fighting for breath during sleep. Morning headache, dry mouth, obesity, excessive daytime sleepiness/involuntary naps may present.
Periodic Limb Movements in Sleep (PLMS) and Restless Legs Syndrome (RLS)	Motor restlessness during sleep and relaxation, involuntary limb movements. Associated with insomnia and/or excessive daytime sleepiness.
Circadian Rhythm Sleep Disorders	Chronobiological disorders involving misalignment between sleep pattern and local time. Delayed or advanced sleep phases produce complaints of insomnia and/or excessive sleepiness.
Narcolepsy	Irresistible sleep attacks at inappropriate times. Sometimes with cataplexy (loss of muscle tone triggered by emotion), hypnagogic hallucinations, sleep paralysis, and disturbed nighttime sleep.
Parasomnias	Abnormal behaviors in NREM sleep (e.g. sleepwalking, sleep bruxism) and REM sleep (e.g. nightmares) and in transition between wakefulness and sleep (e.g. sleep talking).
Sleep Disorders Associated with Medical/ Psychiatric Disorders	A wide range of disorders involves sleep symptomatology. Neurologic disorders (e.g. dementia, Parkinson's disease), other medical disorders (e.g. cardiac ischemia, pulmonary disease, gastrointestinal problems), and mental disorders (e.g. affective disorders, alcoholism).
Extrinsic Sleep Disorders	A wide range of exogenous causes. Includes hypnotic-, alcohol-, and stimulant-dependency sleep disorder.

Source: Based on the revised International Classification of Sleep Disorders, American Sleep Disorders Association, 1997.

the etiology and maintenance of the sleep disorder. The revised version of the International Classification of Sleep Disorders should be consulted for detailed descriptions of the full range of sleep disorders (ICSD-R; ASDA, 1997), however, a brief summary of the major diagnostic categories is presented in Table 3.3. The majority of these has been introduced earlier in the context of specific assessment methodologies. We also draw your attention back to the questions in the latter part of the Sleep History (Table 3.1) because these are designed to help you with differential diagnosis. This section, therefore, will build upon previous information to provide a more complete picture.

Insomnia

As outlined in Chapter 2, the working definition of insomnia is a persistent difficulty initiating and/or maintaining sleep. Sleep-onset or initial insomnia typically comprises greater than 30 minutes of pre-sleep wakefulness (sleep-onset latency; SOL) on the majority of nights, and intermittent or sleep-maintenance insomnia represents 30 minutes of wakefulness from sleep, often accumulated as wake-time after sleep-onset (WASO). The sleep efficiency of insomniacs is usually lower than 85%, that is, they are awake on average for more than 15% of the time they spend in bed. In clinical studies insomniacs typically have more than 60 minutes of SOL and/or WASO and sleep efficiency may be lower than 70%.

Normal Aging

In older people, sleep difficulties must be seen in the context of normal, age-related changes in sleep. Quality, continuity and depth of sleep decline and age-related changes in the circadian rhythm are also observed (Hoch et al., 1997). Differentiating insomnia from normal age-related changes in sleep, therefore, can be problematic. It is a distinction that can only be made clinically, based upon evidence of enduring impact and intrusiveness upon a) sleep itself; b) daytime performance, especially alertness; or c) broader psychosocial functioning e.g. relationships and behavior.

Sleep Related Breathing Disorder (SBD)

SBD refers to respiratory impairment during sleep commonly associated with excessive daytime sleepiness (EDS). Obstructive apneas can be destructive of continuity of sleep, of its restorative powers, and of the experience of sleep quality. Interviewing the partner may provide evidence of respiratory interruption and Epworth Sleepiness Scale scores may be elevated above threshold levels. Lichstein, Riedel, Lester and Aguillard (1999) have recently reported that around one third of their older insomniacs had undiagnosed apneas of clinical significance. This highlights the value of PSG assessment, particularly in older overweight males.

Restless Legs Syndrome (RLS) and Periodic Limb Movement Disorder (PLMD)

The symptoms of these conditions are summarized in Table 3.3 (see also Montplaisir, Nicolas, Godbout, & Walters, 2000). RLS symptoms involve an irresistible urge to move the legs during wakefulness, mostly in the evening, and may significantly delay sleep onset. RLS is primarily a condition of middle to old age, although it is also quite frequent during pregnancy. Nevertheless, in around one-third of cases, symptoms emerge before the age of 20 years (Walters et al., 1996). Similarly, PLMD, which involves muscle twitches in the extremities during sleep, is present more often among older subjects and may be related to disturbance of circadian sleep-wake rhythms in the elderly. Although PLMD may fragment sleep and cause sleep disturbances at night and sleepiness during the day, some patients with frequent periodic limb movements during sleep remain totally asymptomatic. These disorders can be associated with SBD and many people with RLS also experience PLMD. Because the sleep of partners is often interrupted by RLS/PLMD, the partner should be interviewed and the Epworth Sleepiness Scale is also useful. The diagnosis of RLS is made on a clinical basis, whereas PLMD is diagnosed based on PSG assessment, which also provides accurate diagnosis of possible co-existing SBD.

Circadian Disorders

Haimov and Lavie (1997) have reported age-related trends in circadian function. Sleep propensity in young adults was still high at 7 a.m., whereas in elderly people it began to decline at 5 a.m. Older adults also demonstrated increases in sleepiness during the period 7 to 9 p.m. Delayed Sleep Phase Syndrome (DSPS), therefore, is more of a risk factor in younger people and Advanced Sleep Phase Syndrome (ASPS) in later life. DSPS may be confused with sleep-onset insomnia. However, in DSPS, there is less night-to-night variability and subjects remain drowsy for some time if wakened at a normal waking hour, until their internal biological clock signals wakefulness. ASPS is associated with early morning waking, because of the sleep phase advance relative to clock time, and should not be misunderstood as depression unless there are other confirmatory signs and symptoms. Also with advancing age, fragmented sleep can lead to daytime napping, and this further contributes to disorganization of circadian rhythms. Monitoring sleep-wake patterns on a Sleep Diary for two weeks or using actigraphy (cf. Figure 3.2) can assist in the diagnosis of sleep-phase disorders.

Narcolepsy

People with narcolepsy often sleep poorly at night and therefore can present with a symptomatic insomnia. Narcolepsy highlights the importance of a good clinical history. This will generally reveal a peak age of onset of irresistible sleep episodes and EDS at around 15–25 years, with night-time disturbance becoming progressively more problematic with advancing age (Billiard, Besset & Cadilhac, 1983). Patients with suspected narcolepsy/cataplexy should be assessed using PSG and MSLT for diagnostic features such as sleep-onset REM periods.

Parasomnias

Parasomnias are behavioral phenomena occurring during sleep, and may be disorders of arousal, partial arousal or of sleep-stage transition. Although parasomnias normally present first in childhood or adolescence, sudden onset (particularly of REM sleep behavior disorder) in later adulthood may indicate an acute neurological problem (Culebras & Magana, 1987). Parasomnias, however, will seldom be confused with insomnia

Sleep Problems Associated with Medical/Psychiatric Disorders

ICSD-R recognizes that a large number of medical diagnoses may be associated with sleep disturbance. Some examples of common etiologies are presented in Table 3.3. Insomnia may be secondary to illness either because of direct effects upon sleep, or indirectly through pain or discomfort during the night. Medications used to treat illnesses can also impact adversely upon sleep (see below).

Sleep disturbance also features in a wide range of psychiatric disorders, most notably in depression, although there is an association also with other disorders such as panic and generalized anxiety. The differentiation of primary depression from primary sleep disturbance may be best addressed by structured psychiatric interview (Buysse et al., 1997) and through the use of a symptom rating scale for depression. Where insomnia is secondary to depression, other biobehavioral disturbance is usually found e.g. appetite and motivational drive, and negativity in mood is more global and severe, rather than attributed specifically to poor sleep. It is very important to remember, however, that sleep disturbance is one of the most common early signs of the onset of depression (Ford & Kamerow, 1989; Breslau, Roth, Rosenthal & Andreski, 1996), and may persist after depression lifts There is often a failure to recognize the importance of insomnia as a disorder in its own right, and as a risk factor for both first incidence and recurrence of major depressive episodes. PSG assessment may help to differentiate major depression, however, around 50% of depressed outpatients have normal sleep studies. There are, of course, many self-rating scales that permit anxiety and depressive symptoms to be monitored. Of these, the Beck scales (Beck Anxiety Inventory, Beck Depression Inventory), the Hospital Anxiety and Depression Scale, and the Profile of Mood Scales have been most widely used in insomnia research.

Extrinsic Sleep Disorders

Difficulty in initiating and maintaining sleep may result from prescribed drugs, e.g., CNS stimulants, beta-blockers, anti-hypertensives. Useful reviews of this topic are provided by Roehrs (1993) and Roehrs & Roth (2000). Benzodiazepine hypnotics have for long been contraindicated for persistent insomnia due to their adverse effects upon sleep structure and their association with drug withdrawal insomnia (see Chapter 1). Alcohol is the most frequent form of self-medication and is known to worsen sleep disturbance and can exacerbate any existing SBD. Clearly, differential diagnosis requires an accurate history and monitoring of drug use in parallel with Sleep Diary reports.

CLINICAL FORMULATION OF THE SLEEP PROBLEM

In concluding this chapter, we wish to place assessment and differential diagnosis in context. A good sleep assessment will carefully consider possible explanatory hypotheses concerning the etiology and maintenance of the sleep disorder. Valid and reliable assessment may involve subjective and objective methods, and the gathering of information from a partner where appropriate. However, the central purpose of the assessment process is clinical formulation. The interpretation and integration of evidence from these various sources should lead to a working model which guides intervention. An understanding of the impact and intrusiveness of the sleep problem, and appraisal of treatment-related change in these and other target variables, should represent a collaborative agenda for the insomniac and the clinician to follow.

This chapter necessarily has focused upon the assessment of sleep per se, and later chapters will introduce assessment materials that are especially relevant to the selection and implementation of psychological management techniques. The Sleep Hygiene Practice Scale is introduced in Chapter 4, and the Sleep Behavior Rating Scale appears in Chapter 5 in the context of stimulus control treatment. In Chapter 6 on cognitive therapy, three other self-report instruments are presented, namely the Dysfunctional Beliefs and Attitudes about Sleep scale, the Glasgow Intrusive Thoughts Inventory and the Glasgow Sleep Effort Scale. Two more general measures, however, that are long established and widely used, are worth mentioning at this point.

The Pre-Sleep Arousal Scale (PSAS; Nicassio, Mendlowitz, Fussel & Petras, 1985; Appendix E) is designed to quantify separately the somatic and cognitive arousal associated with the pre-sleep period. Although it is specious to think of insomnia in terms of either physiological or mental underpinnings (the two clearly must be inter-dependent), the PSAS nevertheless is a useful tool to identify the predominant pre-sleep experience of the insomniac patient. Similarly, the Sleep Disturbance Questionnaire (SDQ; Espie, Brooks, & Lindsay, 1989; Espie, Inglis, Harvey, & Tessier, 2000; Appendix F) asks the patient to rate a number of possible attributions concerning their inability to sleep. In using the SDQ, physiological, behavioral and cognitive domains can be considered as possible precursors to the insomniac state. Both the PSAS and the SDQ, therefore, can be helpful in determining which components of therapy may be most relevant in a given case. We strongly recommend, however, that our CBT program is delivered in full whenever possible because there is limited evidence supporting the tailoring of therapy as being more effective than applying the best-evidenced intervention plan.

Sleep Hygiene and Relaxation Therapy

INTRODUCTION

In this chapter we will cover two approaches to the management of insomnia that can be conveniently linked together. Components of 'sleep hygiene', and relaxation methods, are often well known to insomniacs because they are commonly reproduced in newspaper and magazine articles as 'simple steps to a good night's sleep'. This is both good and bad. Good in the sense that your patients may already be aware of and interested in behavioral methods; but possibly bad in that they may feel they have already tried everything! You are likely to first become aware of their knowledge and experience when you are taking the sleep history. Certainly, you should make a point of asking about what they have tried before in the way of self-help, and what has worked and not worked. It is useful here to be quite specific, so that you know how exactly they have implemented an idea, and for how long. Remember also that their prior experience is likely to influence their perspective as they start out with you. Some insomniacs arrive at the consulting room with a negative, hopeless mind-set, based in part upon repeated attempts to overcome sleep failure. Others may expect you to come up with something completely novel, and may be disappointed or de-motivated if you rehearse what to them may seem like old ideas. Table 4.1 summarizes some of the factors we think you should have in mind when you start out with a new patient.

We suggest that you use sleep hygiene instructions and relaxation as a starting-point in CBT because, even if people have tried them before, they often have not gained full benefit from what these techniques can offer. We also feel it is a useful experimental test of adherence to see if a

Table 4.1. Factors to Have In Mind When Starting Out with a New Patient

You are probably going to see your patient over a number of sessions to work through the program outlined in this manual. So how are you going to introduce therapy to the patient? There is no absolute way to do this, but we suggest that you bear the following points in mind:

- Patients have often had insomnia for many years.
- They usually have experienced treatment failures.
- These failures may include prescribed medication, over-the-counter products, and behavioral strategies they have read about.
- They may have concerns about sleep medication (eg. don't wish to take drugs; worried about trying to come off).
- They may have felt their complaint of insomnia has not been taken very seriously.
- They may have had difficulty finding someone with expertise to help them.
- Nevertheless, they try to remain hopeful because insomnia is a preoccupying problem.
- They may have other problems, physically and/or mentally.
- Most patients will not have seen a psychologist before.
- CBT is a structured, evidence-based therapeutic approach.
- There is a great deal of evidence supporting clinical effectiveness for persistent insomnia.
- Few patients will have previously used CBT methods systematically, although some components will be familiar.
- CBT is effective delivered by relatively inexperienced therapists providing it is protocol driven, as in using this manual.

patient is able to follow a relaxation routine on a regular basis, or to cut down on caffeine consumption in the evening. Later in our program there will be more demanding suggestions to make! We will explain about sleep hygiene and relaxation in separate sections for ease of understanding.

RATIONALE FOR SLEEP HYGIENE

The term 'sleep hygiene' was first used by Dr. Peter Hauri around 20 years ago to describe what patients themselves can do to eliminate sleep-interfering factors, and to promote good sleep. Sleep hygiene refers to things about lifestyle and preparation for bed that can be changed to improve sleep pattern (see Figure 4.1). You might say that sleep hygiene is good advice for everyone, whether or not they are poor sleepers, and it may be that practicing sleep hygiene as part of a healthy lifestyle might even prevent sleep from sometimes going wrong.

The main lifestyle factors known to have an effect on sleep are caffeine, nicotine, alcohol, diet and exercise. These are primarily stimulants to the central nervous system and liable to promote wakefulness or to interrupt sleep. Even alcohol, which initially acts as a CNS depressant, causes

Lifestyle Factors

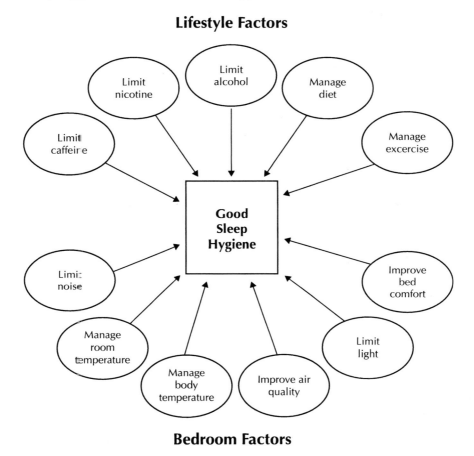

Figure 4.1. Sleep hygiene checker.

wakefulness during the night as its effects wear off. These factors are then largely endogenous. Bedroom factors by comparison are mainly exogenous; to do with how comfortable the bed is, how hot or cold the room is, how well aired, how noisy and how quiet. The idea here is that there is an optimal external environment for sleep. In sleep hygiene, sleep-related lifestyle and the sleep context come together to form a set of sleep-related behaviors that may be more or less suitable for sleep. We find that the Sleep Hygiene Practice Scale (Lacks & Rotert, 1986) is a good way of assessing such sleep-related behaviors. It helps to identify any sleep hygiene problems as well as providing an appraisal of the patient's understanding of such issues. This scale is reproduced in Appendix G as a screening measure for this component of therapy.

Traditionally, sleep hygiene has been regarded as a behavioral insomnia strategy (e.g., Lacks, 1987). However, its components are primarily physiological in terms of a model of insomnia as a disorder of sleep inhibition (Espie, 2002). Excessive caffeine or exercise will delay sleep-onset, presumably through heightened arousal. Indeed, in one experimental study, 400 mg of caffeine three times per day for one week produced increased arousal on metabolic measures and reports typical of insomniac complaint (Bonnet & Arand, 1992). Similarly, environmental factors (temperature, humidity, light) may inhibit sleep physiologically and alcohol may dehydrate or provoke awakenings because of ethanol metabolism. Observing good sleep hygiene, therefore, may remove some potential inhibitors of sleep. Outcome data on sleep hygiene, however, are fairly unimpressive and suggest that it is best regarded as a non-specific component of a more potent intervention package.

PRACTICAL INSTRUCTIONS FOR USING SLEEP HYGIENE ADVICE

You will be able to use the following headings as your checklist for addressing your patient's sleep hygiene needs.

Caffeine

Coffee is not necessarily caffeinated, and caffeine may be in other things as well.

As we explained above, caffeine is a powerful, and readily available, stimulant drug. You should explain to your patients that too much caffeine could be very good at keeping them awake! It is important not to underestimate the effects of a cup of strong coffee. Indeed, an important part of the advice given by road safety authorities internationally to drivers who are sleepy at the wheel is to pull over and have a cup of strong, caffeinated coffee. 200–300 mg. (equivalent to 2 cups of brewed coffee) is sufficient to deter sleep when drivers are sleepy at the wheel.

Most people know that caffeine is found in coffee and tea, but many other products also contain caffeine. For example, cocoa, chocolate bars, carbonated drinks (cola, sodas), 'energy' drinks and over-the-counter analgesics and weight control medicines may contain caffeine. Because caffeine is found in many products, we suggest that you advise your patients to read labels on products they may eat or drink in the evening. Caffeine effects can last for many hours and we suggest that patients should only have de-caffeinated drinks for up to 4 hours before bedtime. We sometimes use a quiz sheet, adapted from an original by Dr. Patricia Lacks, to carry home the message that caffeine is in many products. This is reproduced for your use in Appendix H.

Nicotine

Smoking damages your health; it may also damage your sleep.

Nicotine, found in cigarettes and other tobacco products, is also a stimulant drug and has similar effects to caffeine on sleep. Although many people say that they find that smoking is relaxing, the overall effect of nicotine on the central nervous system is arousal. What this means is that nicotine will generally make it harder to fall asleep, and harder to stay asleep. It may not be the appropriate priority to challenge your patients on their smoking habit, and doing so may deflect attention away from dealing with the insomnia. However, there may be occasions when it is relevant, and information about the counterproductive impact of nicotine upon sleep is probably useful.

Alcohol

The nightcap that doesn't really fit.

Alcohol, unlike caffeine and nicotine, is a drug that depresses CNS function. Normally, depressants should help us sleep, but it has been found that even a moderate amount of alcohol in the evening can have a disruptive effect on sleep architecture and can cause restlessness and wakenings, particularly in the second half of the night (Roehrs, 1993). Alcohol may help your patient to fall asleep at the beginning of the night. It acts in effect like a hypnotic drug. However, as the ethanol is metabolized, withdrawal symptoms may occur causing lighter sleep and arousals. Tolerance to the sedative effects of ethanol may also build up over time, reducing any beneficial effects although its disruptive effects tend to persist. Furthermore, alcohol also contributes toward dehydration. Patients may wake up thirsty, and/or may need to urinate more frequently. For all these reasons, you should advise your patients that you cannot really support the idea of a 'nightcap'! Furthermore, for patients with persistent insomnia, the use of alcohol in an effort to promote sleep is particularly unwise as it can encourage dependence. We recommend that alcohol should be avoided from 4 hours prior to bedtime. Before leaving this subject we would refer you to Chapter 7 where we discuss sleep medications. Taking alcohol to aid sleep is self-medication. There are many parallels between alcohol and hypnotics, not only in terms of pharmacologic action, but also in relation to attribution.

Diet

Don't go to bed on an empty stomach.

Hunger can cause wakefulness. That is why a light snack a little before bedtime can aid sleep. On the other hand, going to bed too full can cause wakefulness. You will be able to use the information provided in the introductory chapter on sleep and sleep processes to explain to your patient that sleep is a very active process. This activity includes the body's metabolism, but it is best not to ask the body to do too much work because this can interfere with sleep continuity. We advise patients to eat only a small amount, if at all, when they wake up in the night.

Dieting to lose weight can also have some effect upon sleep. In particular, weight loss occurring too quickly may lead to broken sleep. You will also recall that heavier people are more likely to snore which can disrupt sleep both for the patient and for others, and may place the patient at greater risk for obstructive airways disease. The most important thing is that you assess whether or not weight contributes to the patient's sleep problem, and advise accordingly.

We also mentioned earlier the importance of patients remaining hydrated. Water is good, but some patients may have tried warm, milky drinks to promote sleep. There is only a small amount of evidence that these are of help in insomnia, but they are certainly preferable to caffeinated drinks or alcohol.

Exercise

Tiring yourself out at bedtime is a bad idea, especially if you are unfit.

People who are physically fit have a better quality of sleep, so a good way to promote sleep might be to encourage patients to exercise three times a week for 20–30 minutes, and to build up their aerobic fitness level. Unfortunately, many people with insomnia are not fit and they take their exercise at the wrong time i.e. last thing before going to bed. They reason, incorrectly, that they will tire themselves out and so will be likely to sleep.

Our advice is that, whereas being fit is beneficial to sleep, people with insomnia should avoid strenuous exercise before bedtime, because this 'wakes up' the nervous system and can lead to problems falling asleep and staying asleep. Even exercise during the evening can have these unwanted effects. To improve nighttime sleep the best time to exercise is in the late afternoon or in the early part of the evening. Walking, swimming, cycling, skating, dancing, squash, badminton, and aerobics are just a few of the many activities that can help. The important thing is to improve general fitness.

We turn now to consider the bedroom itself, and to preparation for going to bed. Noise levels, room temperature, the quality of the air in the bedroom, lighting levels, and the comfort of the mattress and pillows can all influence our sleep.

Noise

Sounds familiar.

Unexpected and sudden noises, if loud enough, will waken most people either from the gentle reverie of the just about asleep stage, or even from deep sleep. The cry of a baby, the sound of a telephone ringing, a car horn and, of course, an alarm clock are all examples of such sounds. However, we get used to noises after a while. For example, people who live near to a railway adapt to the sound of passing trains. Also people tend to get used to noise that is more continuous, like a ticking clock. Nevertheless, it can be that while people may not actually waken in response to noise their sleep may actually be lighter.

Room Temperature

What should be the heat of the night?

Extreme temperatures at either end of the range can affect sleep. A hot room (more than 24° C) can cause restless body movements during sleep, more nighttime wakenings, and less dream type sleep. A cold room (less than 12° C) can make it difficult to get to sleep and can cause more unpleasant and emotional dreams. We recommend room temperature to help promote sleep for most people is, therefore, around 18° C.

Body Temperature

Some like it hot.

People sometimes like to take a hot bath to relax and expect that this will help them to sleep. However, poor sleepers sometimes report feeling warmer than good sleepers. To best prepare for sleep, a bath around two hours before bedtime, rather than immediately before retiring, is best.

Air Quality

All I need is the air that I breathe.

A stuffy room may cause an uncomfortable sleep while fresh air promotes sleep. It is helpful for patients to get the blend of air quality and temperature about right during different seasons.

Lighting

Let there not be light.

Too much light, particularly bright white light, can cause wakefulness. We discussed the role of ambient light in the entrainment of the circadian rhythm in an earlier chapter. We suggest that the bedroom should not be too bright, and a combination of strong street lighting and thin curtains should be avoided. A solution may be to cover windows with thick curtains, blinds or even a blanket. Some people who are sensitive to light, or who have to sleep in the day because of shift work commitments, sleep with blinders on.

Mattress and pillows

What you pay is what you get.

Beds of different qualities have differing life spans. This can be one of those areas where you get what you pay for; and most stores can offer advice. Much is down to personal preference for mattress firmness and pillows.

RATIONALE FOR RELAXATION THERAPY

The conceptualization of insomnia as resulting from physiological over arousal has been around for over 30 years (e.g., Monroe, 1967). Freedman & Sattler (1982) found that, prior to sleep-onset, insomniacs had higher frontalis and chin EMG than good sleepers, however, there is limited evidence of tension reduction as the active mechanism in relaxation therapy, and post-treatment changes in EMG, heart rate or respiration have proven elusive (see Espie (1991), pp. 43–45; Bootzin & Rider (1997) pp. 322–326 for review). Interest in physiological arousal has been rekindled by evidence that insomniacs display neurobiological differences from normal sleepers, such as 24-hour metabolic rate as measured by oxygen use (Bonnet & Arand, 1995). Hyper-arousal has also been investigated in PSG studies where findings consistent with slow wave deficiency accompanied by hyper-arousal of the CNS, suggest that insomnia may result from increased cortical activation (e.g., Merica et al., 1998). Importantly, however, not all objective poor sleepers complain of insomnia, and not all subjective insomniacs have poor sleep (Edinger et al., 2000) suggesting that physiological arousal alone is an insufficient explanation. Other studies have consistently associated cognitive arousal more strongly with sleep disruption, and "having an overactive mind" has been the attribution rated most highly, both by insomniacs and non-insomniacs (Broman & Hetta, 1994; Lichstein & Rosenthal, 1980; Nicassio et al., 1985). Also, Espie et al. (1989) reported that the cognitive items of the Sleep Disturbance Questionnaire (e.g. 'my mind keeps turning things over', 'I am unable to empty my mind') were the most highly rated; findings replicated recently by Harvey (2000a).

Relaxation-based treatments, therefore, may either inhibit autonomic activity and so counteract physiological arousal or, perhaps more likely, facilitate mental (and physiological) de-arousal. Relaxation therapy is moderately effective particularly for initial insomnia (Morin et al., 1999; Chesson et al., 1999) but there is little evidence to suggest differential effectiveness across a range of relaxation methods (progressive muscular relaxation, autogenic training, biofeedback, hypnosis, meditation).

PRACTICAL INSTRUCTIONS FOR USING RELAXATION THERAPY

Bedtime Wind-Down

Getting ready for bed is not just putting on your nightclothes.

You should advise your patients that preparation for a good night's sleep begins earlier than they might think! It is not reasonable to expect simply to fall in to bed at a certain time and to fall asleep. Many people live busy lives, and that busy-ness can lead right up to bedtime. Similarly, why should a good sleep pattern follow on from a disorganized evening schedule? Much of our behavior is in well-rehearsed and 'automatic' sequences—like driving the car. We check the mirrors, signal to move, engage the transmission, check the mirrors again, release the

Table 4.2. Sample Prebedtime Planner

Approximate evening time	Planned schedule	
7:30	Put day to rest using 'Rehearsal and Planning Time' (see p. 97)	**Bedtime wind-down period**
7:45–8:30	Complete work/ household activities of primary importance	
8:30–10:00	Complete other activities	
10:00–11:15	Work/activity completed Relaxation time (reading, TV, relaxation exercises etc.)	
11:15	Pre-bed sequence (lock up, change, wash)	
11:30	Retire to bed Practice relaxation	

brake, and drive away. We suggest, therefore, that people adopt a pre-sleep routine.

Suggest to your patients that their pre-sleep routine starts about 60–90 minutes before bed and encourage them to think through how that time will be occupied and in what order events are best to occur. The idea is not to create a behavioral strait-jacket for them, and make them anxious if they cannot for some reason comply with the pattern. Rather, the objective is to lead them into a sequence of wind-down from the day and readiness for the night. This should after a while become automated and occur fairly much without thought or conscious effort. The sample of a completed planner presented in Table 4.2 is the sort of thing they should be working towards.

Each person's routine will be different, but it is important that a work/activity deadline is set at the start of the plan. This approach is permissive of the very concept of relaxation; a concept that many people are not immediately comfortable with. The time before bed, therefore, may become valuable for your patient, not only as a prelude to sleep, but also in it's own right.

Relaxation Training

Learning to relax is a hard lesson; it can mean changing the habits of a lifetime.

It is not all that difficult to sell to patients the abstract notion that if only they could relax, they would be better able to sleep. It is much harder to get them to the point where they genuinely value relaxation, and they implement a relaxation procedure on a regular basis.

We suggest that you discourage patients from thinking that this is all about a technique, or an audiocassette. We try to get our patients to regard relaxation first as a principle, the principle of "letting go."

1. The "Letting Go" Principle

Relaxing is about giving up, not about striving.

Not everyone engages readily with this principle. Many people with insomnia in fact want to do the opposite—that is, to take hold of the problem, and to sort it out. This perceived need to control sleeplessness may be an expression of a more broadly-based need to control personally-threatening situations; or it may reflect a more specific response to the upset of the insomnia itself. Either way, attempts to control the sleep process are dysfunctional, unnecessary, ineffective and untypical of good sleepers. Letting go, by comparison is a functional response. The technique of paradoxical intention is akin to giving-up trying and we discuss its use in Chapter 6.

2. The Relaxation Goal

Practice makes perfect, or at least better than before.

We know of no evidence that relaxation routines act like a sleeping pill. Patients sometimes expect that they can run through a set of exercises or listen to a tape and it will put them to sleep. Our advice is that you explain relaxation as a training program. That means a learning program; and that means time and practice. Patients should practice under ideal circumstances first of all. Perhaps during the day (but not in the car!) or early evening, when they are not expecting it to make them sleep, but they are able to concentrate on the content. Disciplined, daily daytime practice as well as implementation at night is a good idea. Also explain to patients that the goal of relaxation is relaxation, not sleep, but that sleep is then more likely to follow when the mind and body are relaxed.

3. The Relaxation Method

Being relaxed is the desirable end product; there is more than one way to get there.

We suggest here an abbreviated progressive relaxation program, which involves muscle tension release cycles, breathing control and imagery. However, as we mentioned earlier, there is no evidence for the superiority of one form of relaxation procedure over another. What is important is getting relaxed. A transcript of a relaxation training procedure lasting approximately 12 minutes is reproduced in Table 4.3 and in Appendix I. You may wish to use this transcript to record your own voice on audio tape. This will give you a relaxation master tape that you can copy for your patients. You will then know what they are learning and be better able to deal with their questions.

4. Putting It All Together

In Table 4.4 we have briefly summarized our overall approach to relaxation.

IMPLEMENTATION ISSUES WITH RELAXATION THERAPY

Although patients generally like relaxation exercises, adequate implementation at home should not be assumed. For example, work that has been done using discreet counters, which record how frequently an audio-cassette player has been used, indicate that patients over-report adherence. There are many reasons why patients fail to carry out home assignments, even when they have every intention of doing so. In the case of relaxation, common reasons include not valuing the state of relaxation very highly, feeling guilty when relaxing, and finding it hard to fit in the practice. These reasons have much to do with lifestyle and the patient's expectations of him/herself. It is also common for people to say that they simply forgot. It is worth bearing in mind that any novel procedure is not primed by existing habits, so it is useful to discuss with the patient how and when it will be possible to practice at home. The clinical vignette below illustrates some of these implementation issues.

Finally, at the end of the transcript we mention that the patient may use their 'visualization scene'. You may or may not wish to include this. Imagery techniques are useful for some but not all patients, probably because there are individual differences in the ability to visualize. Of course, this applies also to relaxation in general. Some patients will take to it more

Table 4.3. Transcript of Relaxation Therapy Session (12-Minute Duration)

The exercises on this tape are designed to help you relax. Relaxation is a skill, which you can learn. It is just like any other skill, so don't be surprised if you find it takes practice because that is how we learn skills. So do practice. Practice a couple of times a day, especially as you start to learn. Of course, you will want to use the relaxation when you go to bed, to help you relax and go to sleep, but you will find it most useful if you have already learned what to do.

It is best to practice at a time when you know you won't be disturbed. The tape will last between ten and fifteen minutes so you will need at least that length of time set aside. When you do your relaxation exercises in your bed, you will be able to listen to the tape there too. But after a while you will have learned what to do and you will be able to just follow the exercises in your own mind.

The exercises themselves begin now.

Settle yourself down. Lie down with your hands and arms by your sides; have your eyes closed. That's good.

We will start by just thinking about your breathing. Your breathing can help you relax; the more deep and relaxed it is the better you will feel and the more in control you will feel. So begin by taking some slow regular breaths. Do that now. Breathe in fully, fill up your lungs fully; breathe in, hold your breath for a few seconds now, and let go, breathe out... Do that again, another deep breath, filling your lungs fully when you breathe in, hold it... and relax, breathe out. Continue that in your own time, noticing that each time you breathe in the muscles in your chest tighten up, and as you breathe out there is a sense of letting go. You can think the word 'relax', each time you breath out. This will remind you that breathing out helps you relax. It will also help you to use this word to tell yourself to relax whenever you need to. You will find that your body will begin to respond. Breathing slowly, comfortably, regularly, and deeply; thinking the word 'relax' every time you breath out; enjoying just lying still and having these moments to relax, concentrating on the exercises.

Now, I'd like you to turn your attention to your arms and hands. At the moment just lying at your sides. I'd like you to create some tension in your hands and arms by pressing your fingers into the palms of your hands and making fists. Do that with both hands now. Feel the tension in your hands, feel the tension in your fingers and your wrists, feel the tension in your forearms. Notice what it is like. Keep it going... and now relax. Let those hands flop. Let them do whatever they want to do; just let them relax. Breathing slowly and deeply, you will find that your fingers will just straighten out and flop, and your hands and arms will feel more relaxed. Allow them to sink into the couch or into the bed, just allow your arms to be heavy. Breathing slowly and deeply, thinking the word 'relax' each time you breathe out, and finding that your hands and arms just relax more and more and more. Your arms and your hands so heavy and rested. It's almost as if you couldn't be bothered moving them. Just because you have let go of the energy and tension that was in the muscles there. Breathing slowly and deeply, both your hands, both your arms, heavy and rested. Let go of the energy and tension that was in the muscles there, breathing slowly and deeply. Both your hands, both your arms, heavy and rested and relaxed.

I'd like you to turn your attention now to your neck and shoulders. Again we're going to get your neck and shoulders into a state of relaxation following some tension we're going to introduce. I'd like you to do that by pulling your shoulders up towards your ears. Now, do that; pull your shoulders up towards your ears. Feel the tension across the back of your neck, across the top of your back and in your shoulders. Feel the tension, keep it going not so much that it's sore, but keep it constant. Feel it, and now let go... relax; go back to breathing slowly and deeply. Let that tension drain away,

---

(Cont.)

Table 4.3. (*Cont.*)

---

let it go. Breathe deeply, and as you do so, notice that the tension, almost like a stream, drains away from your neck, across your shoulders, down the upper part of your arms, down the lower part of your arms and out through your fingertips. Draining out and leaving a sense of warmth and relaxation deep in your muscles. Breathing slowly and deeply and allowing that to take place. Just let the tension go. If it doesn't seem to go, don't force it, it will go itself. Be confident about that. Just breathe slowly and deeply and allow yourself to be relaxed; remembering to think the word 'relax', each time you breathe out. Using that word 'relax' to focus on the sense of relaxation that you get, using the word 'relax' to remind you of the success your are having in relaxing your body.

I'd like you to concentrate now on your face, and on your jaw, and on your forehead. I'd like you to create some tension in these parts of your body by doing two things together at the same time. These things are to screw up your eyes really tightly and bite your teeth together. Do these things together now. Bite your teeth together; feel the tension in your jaw. Screw up your eyes; feel the tension all around your eyes, in your forehead, in your cheeks, throughout your face, wherever there is tension. Now keep it going . . . and relax; breathing in through your nose and out through your mouth, slowly and deeply. Notice how your forehead smoothes out and then your eyelids and your cheeks. Allow your jaw to hang slightly open. Allow your whole head to feel heavy and to sink into the pillow; breathing slowly and deeply. Allow there to be a spread of relaxation across the surface of your face and into all those muscles in your face. Allow your eyelids to feel heavy and comfortable, your jaw and your whole head; breathing slowly and deeply, enjoying the relaxation which you feel in your body. Relax each time you breathe out. Relax just that little bit more each time you breathe out.

Concentrating now on your legs and feet, I want you to create some tension here by doing two things at the same time; and these things are to press the backs of your legs downwards and to pull your toes back towards your head. Do these things together now. Create the tension in your legs, press the backs of your legs downwards and pull your toes back towards your head. Feel the tension in your feet, in your toes, in your ankles, in the muscles in your legs. Feel what it is like. Don't overdo it; just notice what it is like . . . and relax. Breathing slowly and deeply once more; just allow your feet to flop any old way. Allow the muscles to give up their energy, give up their tension. Let it go, breathing slowly and deeply. Notice how your feet just want to flop to the side. Notice how your legs feel heavy as if you couldn't be bothered moving them. Heavy and comfortable and rested and relaxed. Just that little bit more relaxed each time you breathe out.

Be thinking about your whole body now; supported by the bed, sinking into it, but supported by it. You've let go the tension throughout your body. Your body feels rested, comfortable. Enjoy each deep breath you take. Just use these few moments now to think about any part of your body that doesn't feel quite so rested and allow the tension to go. It will go. Breathe slowly and deeply; thinking the word 'relax' each time you breathe out. Just let any remaining tension drain away; from your hands, your arms, your neck and your back. Heavy and rested, comfortable and relaxed. From your face and your eyes, from your forehead; letting the muscles give up their energy. Like a stream of relaxation flowing over your whole body. Let your legs and feet feel relaxed; sinking into the bed. Breathing slowly and deeply.

In a few moments, this tape will finish; but you can continue to relax. You may wish to repeat some of the exercises yourself and that is fine. You may wish to enjoy just continuing as your are. You may wish to think on your visualization scene or build pictures in your mind that will help you to relax further. It's up to you, but continue to relax.

The tape itself stops now.

Table 4.4. Your Relaxation Program

Here are the steps you should follow for your relaxation program:

1. Practice relaxation at a convenient time you have set aside
2. Wind down during the second half of the night.
3. Slow down or stop doing work/activity 90 minutes before bed.
4. Practice the relaxation routine while in bed:
   a. Concentrate on breathing as a cue to the relaxation response.
   b. Tense and relax muscles systematically.
   c. Take exercises slowly—do not over tense muscles.
5. Practice, practice, practice.

readily, but there are some particular issues with imagery training. First, we recommend that you try to establish your patient's ability to visualize, and their degree of comfort with the process. You can simply ask them about this or get them to try an experiment in the consulting room. Ask them to close their eyes and try to picture some objects (a boat under sail in a gentle breeze, a clock face with a ticking second hand). See how they get on. Second, it is far better to get patients to decide upon an imaginal scene for them to use during relaxation, than to leave it literally to their imagination at the time. For example, if it is something like walking through a favorite piece of parkland and gardens, they should prepare the scene and the sequence in advance, so it is a bit like 'rolling the tape' when it comes to using the imagery. Finally, we suggest that practice is, once again, very important to train the imagery if it is going to be useful. You might even consider encouraging them to script their scene and you can record it onto the audio tape for them.

CLINICAL VIGNETTE

Although patients generally like relaxation therapy, adequate implementation at home should not be assumed.

THERAPIST: So how are you getting on with the exercises we tried last week?

PATIENT: Fine. I think they do help me relax a bit. Yeah, they're quite good, quite helpful really . . . that's when I remember.

THERAPIST: Tell me a bit more . . . about how you've found them helpful.

PATIENT: Well, I've listened to the tape and it makes a lot of sense . . . to relax more I mean. I'm not good at relaxing, never have been. I feel better after I've done the exercises.

THERAPIST: When have you done them . . . I mean what times? You said about having to remember.

PATIENT: Yes, I haven't been very good . . . but I have done them most days. It's hard to find time during the day or in the evening to practise like you said.

THERAPIST: So, most days are a good start!

PATIENT: Yes, I suppose.

THERAPIST: Do you think there's anything that might make it easier to practise more often?

PATIENT: What do you mean?

THERAPIST: Well, you are saying it's hard to find time . . . and hard to remember.

PATIENT: I just need to make the time I think.

THERAPIST: What time would be best? Is there a time you could set aside?

PATIENT: I should probably be able to manage after dinner, after we've cleared up.

THERAPIST: So that's about when.

PATIENT: Around 7.

THERAPIST: Good. I think if you practised every day around 7 you would learn the program really well . . . probably enjoy it more too, if you've got time set aside.

PATIENT: And I would still use it at night in bed?

THERAPIST: Absolutely. You'd be more likely to benefit because you'd be used to it. Better practised, means more relaxed.

PATIENT: Even if I don't fall asleep doing the exercises I think I'd be less bothered about it.

THERAPIST: I agree. I think to be relaxed about not sleeping would be a big step forward for you.

PATIENT: Yes . . .

Sleep Scheduling

INTRODUCTION

We use the term "sleep scheduling" to describe the synthesis of two components of CBT, namely *stimulus control* and *sleep restriction* therapies. Sleep scheduling can be readily integrated with the sleep hygiene and relaxation procedures introduced in the previous chapter because they are primarily behavioral in their implementation, although the literature suggests that treatment benefit is, at least in part, cognitively-mediated. Successful home compliance is often challenging but these techniques are thought to be amongst the most effective in helping patients with insomnia to improve their sleep pattern.

RATIONALE FOR SLEEP SCHEDULING

We will first consider stimulus control, reflecting it's relatively early emergence in the insomnia literature. Since Dr. Richard Bootzin illustrated the potential application of stimulus control principles using case study material in 1972, an understanding of insomnia as the product of maladaptive sleep habits has had considerable appeal. Good sleep is seen as coming under the stimulus control of the bedroom environment, features of which act as discriminative stimuli for successful sleep (Bootzin, Epstein & Wood, 1991). Difficulty falling asleep may result then either from failure to establish discriminative stimuli for sleep or from the presence of stimuli incompatible with sleep. Examples of the latter include reading, watching television, eating and speaking on the telephone; all essentially waking activities. Poor stimulus control, therefore, might strengthen conditioned arousal in the bedroom and so delay sleep-onset. Similarly, lying awake in bed before getting to sleep, or through the night during wakeful times, may create a learned association between bed and wakefulness. The insomniac may also nap in an armchair and so strengthen associations between sleep and non-sleeping environments. Stimulus control treatment instructions, therefore, comprise lying down to sleep only when sleepy, avoiding using the bed for activities other than sleep (sexual activity excepted), getting up if unable to sleep quickly (within 15–20 minutes), repeating rising from bed as necessary throughout the night, getting up the same time every day, avoiding napping and following all of these seven days per week (Bootzin & Epstein 2000).

However, very few studies have investigated conditioning in insomnia and evidence for this mechanism of effect is, at best, equivocal (see Espie 2002). For example, Harvey (2000a) reported that primary insomniacs did not differ from good sleepers on daytime napping, variable sleep scheduling, whether they stayed in bed or got up when unable to sleep, or on engagement in sleep-incompatible activities. Nevertheless, significantly lower sleep efficiency is typical of insomniacs, and this may evidence the need for improved stimulus control. One of Colin Espie's graduate students recently conducted a study on this and obtained similar results (Harvey & Espie, 2001). In preparation for the study some adaptations were made to an existing questionnaire (Kazarian, Howe & Csapo, 1979) which assesses sleep-related behaviors. You might find this useful so we have reproduced the Sleep Behaviour Rating Scale in Appendix J.

Interestingly, Bootzin has reported that stimulus control reduces sleep anticipatory anxiety as well as improving sleep, which is consistent with our view that stimulus control helps to reduce dysfunctional, sleep-related cognitive activity and enables the insomniac to become less preoccupied and concerned about sleeplessness (Morin 1993; Espie 2002). More research is required because stimulus control interventions have consistently been found to be efficacious (Morin, Hauri et al., 1999). Indeed, they are the only procedures recommended by AASM as comprising 'standard' non-pharmacological treatment for insomnia (Chesson et al., 1999).

Stimulus control also contains an element of temporal adjustment to the sleep pattern and sleep restriction is another technique, which may act both as a circadian harmonic and a reinforcer of homeostatic drive. These terms require a little explanation. Two processes are thought to interact in normal sleep. The sleep homeostat 'drives' the sleep-wake schedule toward a balanced requirement, because prolonged wakefulness builds up 'sleep debt' and sleep pays off the debt, rather like a set of weighing scales; and the circadian timer regulates the biological 'body' clock in approximation to the 24-hour clock (Borbely 1994, Carskadon & Dement, 1981). Sleep restriction addresses inefficiencies and irregularities, which have developed in this

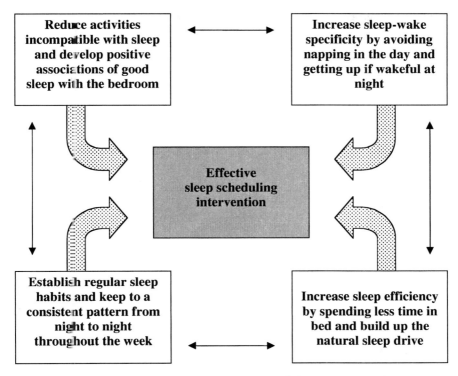

Figure 5.1. Conceptual components of sleep scheduling treatment of insomnia.

schedule to help patients achieve a similar amount of sleep, during the same time period, seven nights per week.

Dr. Art Spielman encouraged his patients to reduce their bedtime hours (by staying up late and/or rising earlier) to approximate time spent in bed more closely to the length of time they were actually sleeping (Spielman, Saskin & Thorpy, 1987). His model of sleep restriction, therefore, compressed sleep toward greater continuity, reduced wakefulness in bed, and increased sleep efficiency. It is important to recognize here that sleep efficiency can be improved either by sleeping longer or by spending less wakeful time in bed. This is an important breakthrough in thinking because insomniacs typically want to sleep longer! However, once sleep pattern is improved, time in bed may be extended, at a rate of 15 minutes per night per week, until the patient no longer gains further sleep and sleep efficiency is at risk of reducing. Wohlgemuth & Edinger (2000) review empirical findings on the efficacy of sleep restriction and AASM support sleep restriction as a 'guideline' intervention for insomnia (Chesson et al., 1999). The latter, limited endorsement, however, reflects the relatively small number of trials that have used sleep restriction alone as a mode of intervention. In clinical practice it is a common component of CBT packages.

The synergy between stimulus control and sleep restriction is evident, and they are often presented together in treatment. As we have said, we use the term 'sleep scheduling' for the combination because there are clear behavioral instructions for the patient to follow which help to establish a regular sleep habit. Figure 5.1 illustrates the ways in which these component processes interact.

PRACTICAL INSTRUCTIONS FOR USING SLEEP SCHEDULING

Objectives

Explain to patients that the purpose of sleep scheduling is to "reshape your sleep so that it meets your individual needs and develops into a strong nighttime pattern".

Insomniacs complain that their sleep is inadequate; that it does not meet their needs. The experience of sleep itself is poor and there are often daytime consequences, such as irritability and concentration problems. Also, they usually complain that they have no real pattern to their sleep but that it varies from night to night. This can make them feel their sleep is out of control. It is important, therefore, that patients understand that the purpose of sleep scheduling is to help them with these very problems. You will also need to motivate them to put the procedures into practice. We will return to the issue of implementation later on. First of all you should have a clear understanding of each of the elements of sleep scheduling. There are quite a few, so we will discuss them one at a time. We have presented them in the sequence that we find clinically to be the most beneficial. You will note, for example, that sleep restriction procedures occur early on because it is our experience that sometimes when the sleep window is reduced, specific stimulus control instructions sometimes become unnecessary or automatic. A summary is presented in Table 5.1 and in Appendix K.

1. Restrict Your Time Spent in Bed

A good starting point is to get whatever amount of sleep you are getting right now all in the one block and the same each night.

Table 5.1. Summary of the Sleep Scheduling Treatment Program

---

1. Work out your current average sleep time and plan to spend that amount of time in bed.
2. Decide on a set rising time to get up each morning and put that into practice.
3. Establish a threshold time for going to be by subtracting sleep time from rising time, and stay out of bed until your threshold time.
4. Lie down intending to go to sleep only when you feel sleepy at or after the threshold time.
5. Follow this program seven days/nights a week.
6. If you do not sleep within 15 minutes get up and go into another room. Do something relaxing and go back to bed when you feel sleepy again. Repeat this if you still cannot sleep or if you waken during the night.
7. Adjust the new schedule by a maximum of 15 minutes per week, dependent upon your sleep efficiency.
8. Do not use your bed for anything except sleep and turn the light out when you go to bed.
9. Do not nap during the day or evening.

Insomniacs often complain of not getting enough sleep, and would like to get more. But perhaps they would not want more of the same! Their sleep is often of poor quality, broken up, and varying from night to night. For example, a person may sleep three or four hours some nights, while other nights manage to get seven. Another common problem is that people waken up during the night, and, although the total number of hours slept may seem okay, if you add all the bits together, wakening up disturbs sleep so that it feels like there were fewer hours. You should explain, therefore, that an important step is to stabilize sleep so that it settles into a pattern that can be relied upon. You should also explain that there will be a better chance of increasing the amount of sleep they get on average once sleep is consolidated into a single block without wakenings. These procedures are part of sleep restriction therapy.

It is hard for your patients to know how much sleep they need right now, especially if the pattern is all over the place. However, you can help them with this by asking them to keep a Sleep Diary and work out an average. Using the diary at Appendix B, ask your patient to keep a record of their sleep for a couple of weeks. Since most of us can manage to divide by 10, it is convenient to use information over a 10-night period to work out the average amount of sleep! You can get them to calculate this by transferring information on total sleep time from the diary to the simple worksheet provided at Appendix L. An illustrative example is provided in the clinical vignette below which accompanies Table 5.2.

Clinical Vignette 1

Mrs. A is a 62-year-old lady who has had insomnia for the past 15 years. She finds that it is problematic to get to sleep, but she also wakens up frequently and her sleep is fragmented across the night. Her sleep diary reveals that she goes to bed most nights at around 11:30 p.m. and rises at 7:00 a.m. In other words, she spends 7 hours 30 minutes in bed. It is evident from the sample of 10 night's of sleep diary data, transferred to Table 5.3, that she does not in fact manage to sleep that length of time; her longest sleep being $6^1/_2$ hours. Furthermore, on two nights she reported sleeping only $3^1/_2$ hours. Her average sleep time over these 10 nights was 5 hours 12 minutes because her estimates of total sleep added to 52 hours. If we then divide Mrs. A's average sleep by her average time spent in bed, and multiply by 100, we can calculate her 'sleep efficiency'. This works out at $(5.2 \div 7.5) \times 100$, which is 69.3%. On average then Mrs. A spends over two-thirds of her time in bed asleep, but importantly, she spends one-third of the night lying awake in bed. This represents her experience of broken, unsatisfying sleep.

The goal of the sleep restriction instruction is to increase sleep efficiency close to 100% by reducing the amount of time spent in bed to approximate to average sleep length. This helps the night's sleep knit back together in a continuous stretch and provides the necessary momentum for sleep duration to expand. The first challenge for Mrs. A then is to spend no more than say $5^1/_4$ hours in bed each night.

We have deliberately chosen an extreme example here to make the necessary points. Please note that we strongly advise that, where patients calculate their average sleep length to be less than 5 hours per night, a duration of 5 hours is used as the default minimum value. There are three reasons for this. First, patients often underestimate how long they sleep; second, the effectiveness of the sleep scheduling program does not depend upon creating sleep deprivation, but upon stabilizing the sleep pattern; and third, this acts as a safety precaution for patients who experience excessive daytime sleepiness.

2. Establish Your Rising Time

Rising at the same time each day acts like an anchor to hold the sleep pattern in the same position.

Your next goal is to help your patient achieve this same amount of sleep each night. An effective way of achieving this is to 'anchor' sleep around an agreed morning rising time. You should explain that this anchoring is to stop sleep from drifting and to help it to settle down into a pattern. Encourage your patient to think of a time to rise each and every morning, including weekends. The time itself is not the most important thing, but it should be one which your patient finds reasonably convenient for the things that he or she needs to do during the day.

Table 5.2. Calculating Current Sleep Requirement for Sleep Restriction

---

First, write down in the spaces below the amount of time you think you actually slept on each
of the last 10 nights, from your Sleep Diary.
Second, add up the total time you have slept across these nights.
Third, divide the total by 10 to get the average length of your night's sleep.

The example below illustrates a variable sleep pattern where the average sleep time is
relatively low (see Clinical Vignette 1).

Night	Amount Slept
1	6 hr 30 min
2	3 hr 30 min
3	5 hr 15 min
4	6 hr 15 min
5	4 hr
6	6 hr
7	5 hr 30 min
8	3 hr 30 min
9	6 hr
10	5 hr 30 min

Total amount of time over 10 days = 52 hr

Average sleep time = 52 hr/10 = 5 hr 12 min

---

3. Establish Your "Threshold Time" for Bed

*When you cross this threshold, it should be time for sleeping right through
the night.*

You now know both your patient's average current sleep requirement
and planned morning rising time. The next thing to discuss is when bedtime should be! Ask how the decision is made about when to go to bed at
the moment.

Sometimes people go to bed before they are sleepy tired and end up
lying awake, or they fall asleep quickly but waken after a short while. This
may occur when an insomniac is trying to 'catch up' on lost sleep, and goes
to bed supposedly for 'an early night'. People sometimes say that they go to
bed because everyone else has gone to bed, or because there is nothing on
television that they want to watch, or just because they feel it is 'bedtime'.
None of these is a good predictor of rapid sleep-onset. People even force
themselves to stay up very late in an effort to exhaust themselves, in the
belief that this will make them sleep better.

The answer to the question, "When should I go to bed?", however,
is fairly straightforward; that is, at a time which makes it likely you will
sleep right through the night. The goal here then is to set what we call

a 'threshold time' for going to bed. This is to mark the point at which your patient can reliably cross the threshold from waking to sleeping. It is worked out simply by subtracting average sleep time from morning rising time.

Here is an example:

>*Average sleep time*:   *6 hr 30 min*
>Set rising time: 7:00 a.m.
>Threshold time: 7:00 a.m. − 6 hr 30 min = 12:30 a.m.

This person sleeps an average of 6 hours and 30 minutes each night and has decided on a morning rising time of 7 a.m. The threshold time for bed then is 12:30 a.m. It will be apparent that there is scope to delay or advance both rising time and threshold time to suit individual preference (e.g., for the sleep time illustrated, a rising time of 6:30 a.m would permit a threshold time of 12 midnight). You should take this into account and plan a personalized schedule with each patient. The important thing is that the patient now recognizes that they have a new 'sleep window' within which they can obtain their night's sleep.

4. Go to Bed Only When You Feel Sleepy

Feeling sleepy is a very important way of telling if you are going to fall asleep.

Your patient needs to be ready to sleep. Tell your patients that it is important that they only go to bed when they think they feel sleepy enough to sleep through the night. If they are not 'sleepy tired' they are more likely to lie awake in bed, and break the connection between bed and sleep. Encourage them to recognize signs such as itchy eyes, lack of energy, aching muscles, yawning and so on, and to respond to these as discriminative stimuli for sleep. Help them also to differentiate tiredness from sleepiness. Tiredness does not mean that sleep is inevitable, whereas sleepiness is a signal from our bodies that it is time for our night's sleep. Importantly, remind your patients that they should not go to bed until they are sleepy *after* their threshold time.

5. Follow a 7-Night-per-Week Schedule

By following the new schedule every single night you will establish a strong pattern for the future.

This is one of the simplest, but also one of the hardest instructions. People often feel that they are 'entitled' to their long lie at the weekend, and may question the need to follow the program so rigidly. Certainly they will express some surprise or even dismay at the 7-night per week rule! However, there are good reasons for encouraging them to persevere. Explain to them that they are engaged in a process of change, which takes some time to have an effect, but which will be accelerated by consistency across the week. The goal is to establish a strong sleep drive and a durable good sleep habit, which will itself be difficult to break once properly established.

6. Observe the 15-Minute Rule

Lying awake in bed is one of the main things that keeps sleeplessness going.

Of course, even when your patient goes to bed sleepy, there will be nights when sleep will not come quickly. You should advise that if sleep does not come within 15 minutes, they should get out of bed and go into another room. After a while of being up, they should go back to bed when feeling sleepy again, but if still unable to sleep, should wait no longer than 15 minutes before getting up once again. This same rule should be applied if your patient has the problem of waking up during the night and has difficulty returning to sleep. The 15-minute rule is one of the hardest for patients to put into practice. If you can encourage a philosophical attitude to not sleeping then that can help, e.g. "I'm not sleeping but just lying here getting frustrated, I might as well get up and come back to bed when I'm properly sleepy".

7. Make Adjustments to Your New Schedule

Building on your success in sleeping more efficiently, you can hope to sleep a bit longer.

Your patients will want to know when they are likely to start to get some more sleep! At first, the idea is that by restricting the amount of time spent in bed your patient will be sleepy enough to sleep right through. Instead of having bits of sleep, sleep becomes consolidated.

But you can explain that there is evidence to suggest that sleep time can continue to increase even months after completion of a CBT program involving sleep scheduling, providing they introduce change systematically. Explain that sleep restriction helps the broken bits of sleep to knit together and that once this has happened the sleep pattern is able to grow to its correct size for that individual.

The practical instruction is to use sleep efficiency as the guiding tool. Once the patient is sleeping 90% of time spent in bed, time in bed can be increased by 15 minutes per night for one week, either by going to bed 15 minutes earlier or by staying in bed this much longer. After this a further check should be made and, if 90% sleep efficiency has again been achieved, a further 15-minute increase in time in bed can be made for the next week. It is important to advise patients not to go beyond 15-minute increments at weekly intervals. Patients may be able to make several of these adjustments, but there will come a time when they are sleeping as much as they need. At that point trying to spend longer in bed will not give them any more sleep. Try to encourage them to settle for that pattern.

Patients may also ask about sleeping longer on weekends. The same principle can apply here. They can examine the efficiency of their sleep on weekend nights. It may be possible for them to sleep longer on weekends than on weekdays and still retain a high sleep efficiency across the week.

8. Make the Connection between Bed and Sleep

Sleep will come more quickly if your mind and body respond to an important cue: your bed.

Your goal is to encourage patients to use their bed only for sleep, so that they build a strong link between bed and sleep. This connection will help promote sleep. This means that activities like watching TV, reading, eating, and talking on the phone are to be kept for other rooms in the house, and banned from the bedroom. Patients should instead be encouraged to put the light out straight away when they go to bed, and put their head down intending to sleep. Sexual activity is the only exception to this rule; it actually helps us sleep afterwards!

9. Avoid Daytime Naps

By cutting out naps you will be better prepared for a continuous, longer sleep at night.

You should explain that another thing to do to strengthen the connection between nighttime sleep and the bed is to avoid napping during the day, and napping in the evening. Certainly, there is evidence that a nap of more than 15 minutes reduces the drive for sleep at night. Stopping all naps provides better preparation for a continuous, longer sleep at night but also strengthens the connection between the bed and successful sleep. Sleeping in a chair in another room weakens that important link and takes time out of the night's sleep.

IMPLEMENTATION ISSUES

Making changes is not easy, even when the changes are likely to help us.

As we mentioned in the introduction to this chapter, home implementation of sleep scheduling can be challenging. Some patients will say that they have tried these procedures before—tried staying up late, tried to get up if they don't sleep, tried not reading in bed, etc. Some may say that they already do some of these things but still can't sleep. In our experience, however, patients have not followed this set of guidelines, and not every night. Once they understand that you are asking them quite literally to follow the program in Table 5.3, they will usually agree that this is something that they have not done before. We want to say a bit about specific issues of adherence and then a bit about motivation in general.

As regards the specifics, we have summarized in Table 5.3 some of our experience of what can work effectively to help patients make plans for implementation and thereby improve compliance and outcome. Hopefully the table is self-explanatory.

Perhaps more than with any other component of CBT for insomnia, sleep scheduling is demanding of behavior change. It is helpful, therefore, also to have some general understanding of motivational issues as they affect human behavior and behavioral change. It is beyond the scope of this essentially practical manual to go into this in any detail, but the take home message is to recognize the need to support and motivate your patients toward effective intervention; the latter requires adherence to the protocol. There are different ways you might try to address motivational issues with your patients and here we present just one that Colin Espie uses in his clinical and research practice. The following text is an extract from a patient handout:

You may have made great efforts in the past to improve your sleep, efforts which have failed. These experiences can make getting motivated to make new changes all the more difficult. Dwelling on these experiences may make it hard for you to try again, and giving up may feel like an easier option. It is important, then, that negative thoughts such as, "I am never going to get a good night's sleep," are replaced with more positive ones like, "This problem is hard to break, but I am going to keep on trying." Keeping motivated is the key to achieving permanent changes in your sleep pattern.

The diagram [Figure 5.2] shows us the process of change. Our motivation can come and go; that is to be expected. Relapses can occur and these are times when you experience a strong feeling of disappointment in yourself and think

Table 5.3. Implementation Issues in Sleep Scheduling Treatment

Component of sleep scheduling	Implementation issues
Restrict your time in bed	Patients often underestimate their sleep on sleep diaries. Working out their current average, therefore, can provide opportunity for reality testing. Often patients are dissatisfied with the amount of sleep they get so they may resist only being in bed for this amount of time. Explain that it is a means to an end. That by learning that they can sleep right through their anxieties about sleep will reduce and their sleep pattern will be more likely to repair itself and grow.
Establish your rising time	Although you generally want to discourage clock-watching, there is no substitute for an alarm call to waken us up! By setting an alarm the patient is committing to a reminder of an agreement within the program. Encourage patients also to tell their partner (if applicable).
Establish your "threshold time" for bed	This may be later than the patient's habitual bedtime. Help the patient to plan how to use any additional time in a pleasurable and relaxing way. Encourage them to be specific about what they are going to do.
Go to bed only when sleepy	Patients, understandably, find it hard to stay up when they are anxious about getting more sleep. Nevertheless, encourage them to remain out of bed and awake until their threshold time. They should treat sleepiness prior to then as occurring within daytime hours and therefore avoid napping.
Follow a 7-night-per-week schedule	Encourage patients to avoid creating exceptions. Weekends are a particular challenge here. Check through sleep diaries with them to verify adherence. Praise their success.
Observe the 15-minute rule	Many patients 'instinctively' want to stay in bed. They may not want to leave the warmth of the bed, or feel they would have nothing to do. Rising may represent failure, or cause worry that it would disturb others. Encourage them to expect to be up and so to make a specific plan e.g. leave the heating and a lamp on in the living room, prepare a flask of a warm milky drink or a decaffeinated drink before going to bed, leave some music or a book on the table. Remind them that they can go back to bed when they feel sleepy again.
Make adjustments to the schedule	Patients may be keen to increase time in bed too rapidly. Emphasize gradual change (15 min per week maximum). Encourage them to be their own scientists by calculating sleep efficiency.
Make the connection between bed and sleep	It may be difficult for patients to give up valued habits, which they may report as pleasurable or 'normal behavior'. Encourage them to enjoy these activities, but in a different room, before going to bed, because your goal is to achieve rapid sleep-onset once in bed.
Avoid daytime naps	Many patients already know to try not to nap. Reinforce this with them because the sleep scheduling program can be difficult. For those who do nap, deal with their rationalizations by explaining that the goal is to build up the sleep drive for night-time. Discuss the differences between resting and napping.

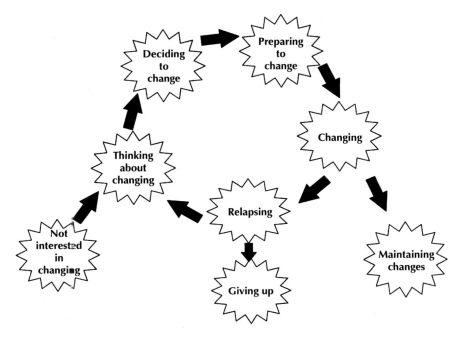

Figure 5.2. Considering readiness to implement parts or all of the sleep scheduling program using the process of change model.

that there is no point in trying again. Please don't let relapses discourage you. The best thing to do is to get right back on that horse and try again! You may never have a better chance to sort out your sleep problems than now

The diagram, which is a version of Prochaska and DiClemente's stages of change model can be used in the consulting-room session to work through general and specific implementation obstacles, like those that might be associated with components of sleep scheduling.

The following clinical vignettes also illustrate some of the implementation issues with sleep scheduling treatment, and how to address these.

Clinical Vignette 2

In this scenario the patient appears reluctant to implement a new schedule which involves sleeping within the planned "sleep window."

PATIENT: So you are asking me to stay up later *and* to get up earlier

THERAPIST: That's what seems to be necessary if we are going to get your sleep back in proper shape . . . so that you can sleep right through

PATIENT: And I'm not supposed to go to bed until midnight and to get up 6.30 every day?

THERAPIST: You could make it 12:30 and get up at 7 if that would be better . . . as long as your sleep window is $6^1/_2$ hours

PATIENT: But I've tried this before

THERAPIST: Tried what?

PATIENT: Staying up late. It didn't work. I thought if I tired myself out I'd sleep OK but I just got all wound up

THERAPIST: Do you think things always work the first time you try them?

PATIENT: What do you mean?

THERAPIST: Because you tried it before you are scared the same thing will happen again? But maybe that's not right . . . and you would need to stick at it to see if it really works

PATIENT: It's such a horrible thing, not sleeping I mean. I hate it

THERAPIST: I agree . . . that's why you're here. I guess I'm thinking that your sleep pattern is pretty bad, and that it needs this amount of work. It isn't really sorting itself out at the moment

PATIENT: I know, I know. I suppose I should give it a try. So if I go to bed at midnight . . .

THERAPIST: . . . any time after then as long as you feel sleepy

PATIENT: Yeah. I can maybe read in the living room

THERAPIST: Good idea

PATIENT: And get up the same time . . . at 6:30. Every day?

THERAPIST: Yes, including weekends

PATIENT: For how long?

THERAPIST: For as long as it takes . . . to get you sleeping through

PATIENT: You really think that will happen

THERAPIST: I'm pretty sure you can do it if you make your mind up . . . and then we'll see how you sleep

PATIENT: It's going to be hard, but I'll do it

THERAPIST: Insomnia is a hard problem to crack . . . but this is the way to crack it.

PATIENT: OK, that's my challenge for this week!

Clinical Vignette 3

In this scenario the patient is being encouraged to implement the 15-minute rule.

THERAPIST: The 15-minute rule means that you won't have long spells lying awake in bed. Instead, you get up and go back to bed when you feel sleepy again

PATIENT: 15 minutes doesn't seem very long to give yourself to fall asleep

THERAPIST: Well, I understand that. You are taking such a long time right now...but really we want to establish rapid sleep-onset in bed. That's why I recommend 15.

PATIENT: What if I'm lying there nice and relaxed...maybe just about to fall over? Besides I might waken my husband if I get up and that's not very fair to him

THERAPIST: It's good if you can be relaxed, but if you were relaxed and sleepy tiredness was on you, you probably would have fallen over quicker than 15 minutes. Does your husband fall asleep before you do?

PATIENT: As soon as his head hits the pillow he's out like a light. It's infuriating!

THERAPIST: So he falls asleep quickly then? That's what we're aiming at for you too...Does he know you are coming to see me?

PATIENT: Yes, thinks it's about time I got this thing sorted out

THERAPIST: Sounds like he might understand you having to get up for a while...if it's going to help

PATIENT: Yes, I suppose so...

THERAPIST: And if you tell him what you're trying to do it might stop you worrying about disturbing him.

PATIENT: I think that's right. It's more that I'm worried about it. It wouldn't bother him, he'd probably sleep right through!

THERAPIST: And I think you said 'infuriated'...that he's so good at sleeping and you're not?

PATIENT: Yes, that too

THERAPIST: Well, the 15-minute rule stops all that because you just make up your mind to get up

PATIENT: Do I have to do it exactly. I don't want to start watching the clock. That would make me worse

THERAPIST: Good point! Absolutely not. Just make it around 15 minutes...as an estimate. You can turn the clock away from you if it's a problem

PATIENT: OK...well I'll speak to my husband when I get home and start this tonight

THERAPIST: Well done. Now let's just have a think about what you might do when you get up...because it will probably happen tonight and it's best to be prepared...

Cognitive Therapy

INTRODUCTION

Cognitive therapy is a psychotherapeutic method designed to change a person's beliefs, expectations, appraisals, and attributions. In the context of insomnia, cognitive therapy seeks to change sleep expectations, perceived causes and consequences of insomnia, and beliefs about sleep-promoting practices. Since its initial formulation by Aaron Beck, cognitive therapy has been adapted to a variety of clinical problems including depression, anxiety, substance abuse and, more recently, to insomnia. This chapter reviews practical applications of cognitive therapy to insomnia. After discussing the role of dysfunctional cognitions in insomnia, the rationale and objectives of cognitive therapy are outlined, practical strategies for changing faulty beliefs and attitudes about sleep are reviewed, and clinical vignettes are presented. As we shall see, this intervention is predominantly verbal in nature and is more time consuming to implement than behavioral procedures described in previous chapters. Nonetheless, it is often a critical component to the successful management of insomnia. We will conclude this chapter with a brief description of other cognitive techniques that can also be helpful in treating insomnia (e.g., paradoxical intention).

THE ROLE OF DYSFUNCTIONAL COGNITIONS IN INSOMNIA

Insomnia is often precipitated by stressful events such as a change of employment, a separation, medical illness, or bereavement. Sleep usually normalizes after the stressor has faded away or the person has adapted to its more enduring presence. For some individuals, perhaps those who are

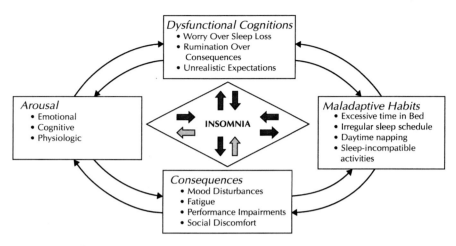

Figure 6.1. The vicious circle of persistent insomnia. *Source*: C.M. Morin (1993). *Psychological assessment and management.* New York: Guilford Press. Reprinted with permission.

more vulnerable to insomnia, sleep disturbances may develop a chronic course. The individual responses to the initial sleep difficulties, mainly his or her behaviors and thoughts, determine in large part whether the sleep disturbance will cease or develop a chronic course. Insomnia is more likely to persist over time if a person interprets this situational insomnia as a sign of danger or loss of control and begins to monitor sleep loss and to worry about its consequences. As shown in Figure 6.1, these types of cognitive responses (e.g., worrying, unrealistic expectations, faulty appraisals) may become dysfunctional and feed on the vicious cycle of insomnia, emotional distress, and more sleep disturbances. Such a chain reaction produces a state of hyperarousal (physiological and emotional), which is literally opposite to the relaxation state required to sleep. We have already addressed (chapter 5) the influence of maladaptive habits on insomnia as well as behavioral strategies to curtail those behaviors. The present discussion will focus on beliefs and attitudes and the use of cognitive strategies to treat insomnia. Whether the main intervention is behavioral or pharmacological in nature, it is essential to address directly the patient's underlying beliefs regarding sleep and insomnia. For instance, even if a patient agrees to reduce the amount of time spent in bed in order to improve sleep continuity, he or she may continue to experience sleep disturbances unless the underlying concerns about the consequences of sleep loss have also been addressed in treatment.

There are two lines of evidence supporting the role of cognitive factors in insomnia. Some studies have focused on intrusive thoughts at night and others have examined the underlying and, perhaps, more affectively laden beliefs and attitudes about sleeplessness that takes place during the day as well as at night. Individuals with insomnia tend to report more negative thoughts about sleep and other themes (health, work, family) during the pre-sleep period and during nocturnal awakenings than good sleepers (Fichten et al., 1998; Harvey, 2000b; Watts, East & Coyle, 1995). Negative cognitions about sleep (e.g., thoughts about not falling asleep) during the period preceding sleep onset are associated with longer subjective sleep latency (Van Egeren, Haynes, Franzen, & Hamilton, 1983). In addition, insomniacs tend to engage more frequently than good sleepers in self-monitoring activities (clock watching, body sensations) and in safety behaviors (calculating time left to sleep) (Harvey, 2000b). Whether this cognitive activity causes insomnia or simply represents an epiphenomenon of wakefulness remains unclear.

Other research indicates that the content and affective tone of sleep-related cognitions may play a greater role in mediating insomnia than the rate of cognitive activity alone. Increasing evidence suggests that dysfunctional beliefs and attitudes about sleep are instrumental in producing insomnia. For example, individuals with persistent insomnia tend to endorse more frequent and stronger dysfunctional beliefs and attitudes about sleep than self-defined good sleepers (Morin, Stone, Trinkle, Mercer, & Remsberg, 1993). Specifically, poor sleepers held more unrealistic expectations about their sleep requirements, stronger beliefs about the consequences of insomnia, and worried more about losing control and about the unpredictability of sleep than normal controls. In addition, these same dysfunctional cognitions have been associated with greater emotional distress and more severe insomnia complaints (Edinger et al., 2000). Recent studies have also shown that changes in those cognitions may actually mediate sleep improvements (Edinger, Wohlgemuth, Radtke, Marsh & Quillian, 2001a; Espie, Inglis, Tessier & Harvey, 2001; Morin, Blais & Savard, 2002). Collectively, these findings tend to support clinical observations that erroneous beliefs and misconceptions about sleep are instrumental in producing emotional arousal and sleep disturbances and should be targeted in the management of insomnia. These cognitions are probably more deeply ingrained than automatic thoughts and are likely to take place, not only at night, but equally during the day.

Based on these two lines of evidence, some authors have used interventions aimed at controlling intrusive thoughts at bedtime with procedures such as imagery training, worry control, and thought stopping, whereas others have used cognitive restructuring therapy to alter dysfunctional beliefs and attitudes about sleep. The next section will focus on this latter approach which targets affectively laden cognitions rather than automatic-intrusive thoughts.

RATIONALE AND OBJECTIVES

Cognitive therapy is based on the assumption that negative emotions, maladaptive behaviors, and physiological symptoms associated with psychological disorders are largely the result of dysfunctional cognitions (Freeman, Pretzer, Fleming & Simon, 1990). The term dysfunctional cognition is used to describe faulty or distorted beliefs, expectations, appraisals, or attributions. Hence, a person becomes anxious or depressed, not because of the external events or the outside world, but because of his or her own perceptions and interpretations of those events. Likewise, a person may experience sleep disturbances because of real stressful events, but such difficulties are typically exacerbated because of the person's appraisal of insomnia and its consequences. Accordingly, the primary goal of cognitive therapy is to guide patients to re-evaluate the accuracy of their thinking and to re-interpret events and situations they experience in a more realistic and rational way. In the context of insomnia, cognitive therapy seeks to alter dysfunctional beliefs and attitudes about sleep in order to decrease emotional arousal and to promote sleep. This is accomplished by guiding the patient to identify maladaptive sleep cognitions, challenging their validity, and reframing them into more adaptive substitutes. The main targets of cognitive therapy are:

- unrealistic expectations about sleep needs and daytime functioning
- misconceptions and false attributions about the causes of insomnia
- distorted perceptions of its consequences
- faulty beliefs about sleep-promoting practices

The objective of therapy is not to deny the presence of sleep difficulties or minimize their impact on a person's life. Rather, it is to guide patient to view insomnia and its consequences from a more realistic and rational perspective. Also, because patients often perceive themselves as victims of insomnia, an important goal of therapy is to strengthen their sense of control and coping skills for managing sleep difficulties and their daytime consequences.

PRINCIPLES AND PRACTICE OF COGNITIVE THERAPY

Cognitive therapy is a structured and directive psychoeducational intervention that relies on a variety of procedures such as reappraisal, reattribution, decatastrophizing, attention shifting, and hypothesis testing. As a preliminary step to implementing cognitive therapy, it is important to provide patients with a brief explanation of the role of cognitive factors on their insomnia. It is often easier to start off with examples, unrelated to insomnia, which can trigger various negative emotions (e.g., being stuck in a traffic jam; not being selected for a job). The important point is to illustrate how a person's interpretation or appraisal of a given situation modulates the types of emotional reaction to that situation. Collaboratively, the clinician and the patient elicit several examples to illustrate this relationship between thoughts, emotions, and behaviors. Once the rationale is understood and the importance of targeting beliefs and attitudes about sleep is integrated, the next steps are to identify patient-specific dysfunctional sleep cognitions.

Identifying Dysfunctional Sleep Cognitions

A most important task is to identify the patient's dysfunctional thoughts about sleep. Many patients are unaware of these thoughts and of their influence on the development of anxious or dysphoric emotions fueling their sleep disturbances. Thus, increasing awareness of those cognitions is a crucial component of treatment. Self-monitoring is usually the most effective strategy to achieve this goal. Because of their automatic quality and inconspicuous nature, training is often essential to help patients obtain adequate records of their thoughts. It is important to point out to patients that these self-statements continually flow through their mind in response to external events (e.g., a bad night's sleep, poor work performance). Although not everyone engages in this process to the same extent, virtually every person who experiences sleep disturbance entertains some thoughts about the causes and consequences of poor sleep.

Starting from a recent example when the patient had trouble sleeping, the therapist guides the patient to identify the automatic thoughts and the associated emotions. The therapist can ask questions such as, "What was running through your mind when you were unable to sleep? How did you feel at that time?" The patient may also be asked to imagine himself or herself in a distressing situation and to report thoughts and emotions triggered by that situation.

> THERAPIST: Close your eyes and listen carefully to this. It's 3:00 AM, and you have been tossing and turning for the past two hours, but nothing seems to help you get back to sleep. You keep wondering whether you'll ever go back to sleep. You worry about all the work you have to do tomorrow. Now, tell me what goes through your mind right at this moment.
>
> PATIENT: Well, I feel that I'm getting uptight and tense. No matter how hard I try to go back to sleep, nothing seems to work. I have to get back to sleep pretty soon; otherwise, I'll be a mess tomorrow. I've

got only three hours left before getting up. If I don't get back to sleep soon, I know I'll feel miserable and won't be able to function at work tomorrow.

Along with verbal questioning and imagery recollection, it is most helpful to use a daily record of automatic thoughts about sleep and insomnia. Table 6.1 presents an example of this daily record with the standard three-column format (see also Appendix M). The patient is asked to identify (1) the situation or activating event, which may involve a stream of thoughts, daydreams, or recollections that led to the unpleasant emotion, (2) the automatic thoughts and/or image(s) that went through his/her mind at that time, and (3) the emotional reactions (e.g., helplessness, anxiety, anger). The intensity of his/her emotional reactions is rated on a scale from 0 to 100. Patients should keep this record on a daily basis and pay particular attention to their automatic thoughts when they have trouble sleeping at night or functioning during the day or, simply when they worry about sleep. The more consistent a patient is in keeping this record, the easier it will be to identify his or her faulty thinking about sleep, and the easier it may be to correct it during therapy.

Another useful method to identify some of the patient's sleep cognitions is *The Dysfunctional Beliefs and Attitudes about Sleep Scale* (DBAS) (Morin, 1994). The DBAS is a 30-item self-report scale (see Appendix N) designed to assess sleep-related beliefs and attitudes. The patient indicates to what extent he/she agrees or disagrees with the statement on a 0 (strongly disagree) to 10 (strongly agree) Likert-type scale. The reader can refer to the appendix for scoring and interpretation guidelines. For now, simply consider that there are no right or wrong answers; rather, their dysfunctional nature is reflected by the degree with which patients endorse a particular statement. The content of those items reflects several themes described previously, such as sleep requirement expectations, causal attributions and perceived consequences of insomnia, control and predictability of sleep, and beliefs about sleep-promoting practices

Table 6.1. Example of a Self-Monitoring Form of Sleep-Related Thoughts

Situation	Automatic thoughts	Emotions
Watching TV in the evening	"I must have some sleep tonight, I have so much to do tomorrow."	Anxious, 80%
Lying in bed awake at 4:00 a.m.	"I have to find a way to get over this sleep problem."	Helpless, 90%
Unable to accomplish tasks efficiently at work	"I knew this would happen after such a poor night's sleep."	Irritable, 60%

Table 6.2. Selected Items from the Dysfunctional Beliefs and Attitudes about
Sleep Scale

Causal attributions of insomnia

   I believe insomnia is essentially the result of a chemical imbalance.

Perceived consequences of insomnia

   I am concerned that chronic insomnia may have serious consequences for my physical
   health.
   After a poor night's sleep, I know that it will be interfering with my daily activities on the
   next day.
   When I feel irritable, depressed, or anxious during the day, it is mostly because I did not
   sleep well the night before.

Sleep requirements expectations

   I need 8 hours of sleep to feel refreshed and function well during the day.
   Because my bed partner falls asleep as soon as his or her head hits the pillow and stays
   asleep through the night, I should be able to do so too.

Control and predictability of sleep

   I can't ever predict whether I'll have a good or poor night's sleep.
   I am worried that I may lose control over my abilities to sleep
   My sleep problem is getting worse all the time and I don't believe anyone can help

Beliefs about sleep-promoting practices

   A "nightcap" before bedtime is a good solution to sleep problems.
   When I have trouble getting to sleep, I should stay in bed and try harder.

(see selected items in Table 6.2). Although this scale was designed initially
to evaluate the severity of dysfunctional sleep cognitions, it is also a very
useful tool for clinicians to identify and select relevant targets for cognitive
therapy sessions.

   The DBAS is administered as part of the initial evaluation with other
self-report measures (e.g., Insomnia Severity Index). For cognitive therapy purposes, you should highlight those items for which the patient's
responses fall towards the upper quartile (i.e., tend to strongly agree with
the statement). Again, while there is no right or wrong responses, the assumption is that a patient would benefit from changing his views or beliefs
on those particular items. Another useful tool is the Glasgow Content of
Thoughts Inventory (GCTI: Harvey & Espie, in press). The GCTI is reproduced in Appendix P. This instrument is derived from extensive work
identifying the 'live' cognitions that insomniacs have while lying awake in
bed unable to sleep (Harvey & Espie, in press; Wicklow & Espie, 2000). It
is, therefore, a valid assessment of the nature of intrusive thought content
and you may find it helpful to appraise your patient's pre-sleep thinking.

Table 6.3. Examples of Probing Questions

---

1. What is the evidence that supports this idea?
2. What is the evidence against this idea?
3. Is there an alternative explanation?
4. What is the worst that could happen? Could I live through it?
5. What is the best that could happen?
6. What is the most realistic outcome?
7. What would I tell _____ (a friend) if he or she were in the same situation?
8. How would someone else interpret the same situation?

Source: J. Beck (1995). *Cognitive therapy: Basics and beyond.* New York: Guilford Press. Reprinted with permission.

Challenging Dysfunctional Sleep Cognitions and Changing Them with More Rational Substitutes

Once patient-specific sleep cognitions are identified, their validity should be examined. The main task is to encourage the patient in viewing his/her thoughts as only one of many possible interpretations, rather than absolute truths. A variety of probing questions is suggested to guide the patient to check the validity of those cognitions (see Table 6.3). Then, the next step consists of finding alternatives to the dysfunctional cognitions by using cognitive restructuring techniques. Self-monitoring is still very useful at this stage to help the patient modify his/her thinking about sleep and realize how much the emotional reaction changes depending on the nature of the thoughts entertained. For that purpose, two columns are added to the daily record of automatic thoughts. First, more rational and realistic thoughts are identified and, second, the associated emotions are re-assessed as a function of this alternative thinking (see Table 6.4).

There are several cognitive restructuring techniques that can be used to challenge and reframe maladaptive cognitions. These include such

Table 6.4. Example of an Automatic Thought Record Used for
Cognitive Restructuring

Situation	Automatic thoughts	Emotions	Alternative thoughts	Emotions
Awake in bed in the middle of the night	"I won't be able to function tomorrow"	Anxious, 80%	"There is no point in worrying about this now. Sometimes I can still function after a poor night's sleep".	Anxious, 25%

techniques as reappraisal, reattribution, decatastrophizing, attention shifting, and hypothesis testing. While it is beyond the scope of this chapter to describe those techniques in details, we will illustrate their utilization in the clinical vignettes presented below. For more information about cognitive therapy procedures, the reader can refer to other sources (Beck, J., 1995; Freeman et al., 1990; Padesky & Greenberger, 1995).

PRACTICAL RECOMMENDATIONS FOR CHANGING BELIEFS AND ATTITUDES ABOUT SLEEPLESSNESS

Keep Realistic Expectations

There is a widespread belief that 8 hours of sleep is a necessity to feel refreshed and function well during the day. Likewise, some people come to expect that they should always wake up in the morning, feeling completely rested and full of energy. Concerns and worries may arise when such expectations are not met. There are individual differences in sleep needs and short sleep is not always abnormal. Also, daytime energy fluctuates from day-to-day, even among sound sleepers. The main message to communicate to your patient is that if they are not feeling completely rested or some days, it is not necessarily abnormal, nor does it always mean that their sleep was disrupted the night before. Urge them to avoid placing undue pressure on themselves to achieve certain gold standards (e.g., 8 hours of uninterrupted sleep), as this is likely to increase performance anxiety and perpetuate sleep disturbances. To determine optimal sleep duration, ask your patient to experiment with various durations and check how they are doing the next day. They may already have done that with the sleep scheduling (sleep restriction) procedure.

Revise Attributions about the Causes of Insomnia

There is a natural tendency to attribute one's sleep problem to external factors (e.g., chemical imbalance, pain, ageing), which a person may have little control over. Although those factors may contribute to sleep disturbances, the exclusive attribution of insomnia to such external causes is likely to reinforce the underlying belief that nothing can be done to improve sleep, that the patient is a helpless victim. You should encourage your patient to adopt a more productive thinking; while it is appropriate to recognise the role of these external causes, it is also essential to identify other factors over which they may have some control (e.g., irregular sleep scheduling, napping, spending excessive amounts of time in bed).

Insomnia is a complex problem and unidimensional explanations should be replaced by multidimensional ones.

Don't Blame Sleeplessness for All Daytime Impairments

Many individuals blame insomnia for everything that goes wrong during the day—fatigue, irritability, and concentration problems. Although poor sleep may indeed produce some of these consequences, the exclusive attribution of all daytime impairments to insomnia is erroneous and, ultimately, perpetuates the insomnia course. So, ask your patients to raise the following question: "Could something else bother me and affect my daytime functioning?" Most likely, they will find that they worry about other things in life (e.g., relationships, work, health) which may affect their mood and reduce their energy. Guide your patient to examine other possible sources of daytime impairments. Once again, it is important to recognize that insomnia does, indeed, have a negative impact on daytime functioning and quality of life. However, it is equally important not to have a single explanation for those deficits.

Don't Catastrophise after a Poor Night's Sleep

Sometimes worrying turns into catastrophic thinking. Some patients are concerned that insomnia may have serious consequences on their health, others consider that not sleeping well deteriorate their physical appearance, and still others see insomnia as an indication of complete loss of control in their lives. Quite frankly, it is often those types of concerns about the perceived/potential consequences of insomnia, rather than the sleep problem per se, which prompt patients to seek treatment. Check with your patient to see if there is a tendency to exaggerate the real impact of insomnia on his or her life? If so, always place things in perspective and ask them "What is the worst that can happen if you don't sleep tonight? Also, remind them that insomnia can be very unpleasant but it is not necessarily dangerous!

Don't Place Too Much Emphasis on Sleep

Some individuals reduce significantly their activity level because of poor sleep and lack of energy. For those people, sleep is the essence of their existence. Their entire life is organised around their sleep—social, occupational, and family activities are contingent upon sleep quality and duration. If sleep is disrupted on a given night, they call in sick or cancel scheduled commitments. Unless sleep improves, these individuals feel they can no longer enjoy life and keep up with their obligations and leisure activities. Check to see if your patient does that. If so, it only gives them more time to dwell on the fact they have not slept well the night before and to worry about the upcoming night. Although sleep occupies one third of our lives, and is an essential ingredient of good quality of life, ask your patient not to give it more importance than it deserves and to resume their daily activities. In this attention-shifting process, it may be necessary to challenge some of the reasons for reducing activities or social contacts with friends and family members. Sometimes, secondary gains or even depression may become an additional focus of treatment. Although it is important for the clinician to show empathy for those people, at the same time, it is equally important to bring them to stop viewing themselves as a victim of something they have no control over.

Develop Some Tolerance to the Effects of Sleep Loss

Instead of dwelling on insomnia and its negative effects on daytime functioning, a more productive approach is to develop some tolerance to sleep loss. Encourage your patient to go on with their daily routines and activities, even after a poor night's sleep. Not easy, but it will shift the focus of their attention away from sleeplessness; it may even convince them that daytime functioning is not entirely dependent upon the previous night's sleep. A useful experiment is to instruct your patient to schedule a pleasant activity specifically after a poor night's sleep in order to disconfirm the view that sleeplessness prevents him or her from doing what he/she wants to do.

Never Try to Sleep

Trying to force sleep is the worst mistake one can make because sleep cannot be achieved on command. Although a person may keep himself awake, up to a certain point, it is simply impossible to induce sleep at will. Whenever a person tries too hard to control or to accomplish something, it backfires and impairs performance—the classic performance anxiety. Explain to your patient that all he can do to promote sleep is to create favourable circumstances and to just let it come. Sometimes, it may even be useful to simply try to stay awake in order to create a paradox (i.e., paradoxical intention) and sleep may just come faster!

These practical and straightforward recommendations may be sufficient for some patients to change their beliefs and attitudes about sleep and insomnia. For others, it may be necessary to rely on more sophisticated cognitive restructuring techniques to get the message across.

Table 6.5. Cognitive Strategies for Changing Beliefs
and Attitudes about Sleep

- Keep your expectations realistic.
- Examine your attributions about the causes of insomnia.
- Do not blame all daytime impairments on sleeplessness.
- Do not catastrophize after a poor night's sleep.
- Do not give too much importance to sleep.
- Develop some tolerance to the effects of sleep loss.
- Never try to sleep.

Implementation of some of those techniques is illustrated in the following clinical vignettes.

CLINICAL VIGNETTES

This section presents three clinical vignettes to illustrate how to implement cognitive therapy using a patient's responses to the DBAS scale.

Vignette 1

In the first scenario, the therapist is attempting to challenge and correct some unrealistic expectations about sleep needs and daytime energy.

"I must have 8 hours of sleep every night to feel rested and function well during the day"
"I should always arise in the morning feeling well-rested"

THERAPIST: Some of your responses on the beliefs and attitudes questionnaire suggest that you feel quite strongly about the need for 8 hours of sleep every night.
PATIENT: Well, I've always thought that we need 8 hours of sleep to stay healthy.
THERAPIST: Many people think like you and, to some extent, you are right.
PATIENT: Isn't it abnormal to sleep only 6.5 hours per night?
THERAPIST: Not necessarily! The important point here is to realize that there are individual differences in the amount of sleep we need to feel rested and function well during the day. As an analogy, do all people you know have the same height?
PATIENT: Of course not!
THERAPIST: What is the normal height for an adult?
PATIENT: Well, there is no norm that applies to everyone. It varies....

THERAPIST: It is similar for sleep. Although most people report about 7 or 8 hours of sleep, some can get by with less and still feel rested in the morning. It is possible that 6.5 hours of uninterrupted sleep be more satisfying and refreshing than 8 hours of broken sleep. So, it will be important to experiment with various sleep durations to determine what is the optimal duration for you. Pursuing unrealistic goals is counterproductive and may actually make you anxious and, as a consequence, perpetuate the underlying sleep difficulties.

THERAPIST: I also noted that you are very concerned when you are not fully rested in the morning.

PATIENT: Well, this concerns me because I assume that if I am not well rested in the morning, it must mean that I have not slept well the night before.

THERAPIST: This may be a valid assumption. However, even the best sleepers do not always arise in the morning feeling well-rested and full of energy.

PATIENT: So, you're telling me that when I wake up in the morning feeling tired, it is not necessarily an indication of poor sleep.

THERAPIST: What I am suggesting is that you need to be careful with your expectations and interpretations. Even with good quality sleep, you simply cannot expect to always feel refreshed and energetic during the day. There are day-to-day variations in how we feel and how energetic we are.

PATIENT: I guess I have noted that for myself.

THERAPIST: So, what alternative thoughts should you have the next time you catch yourself setting standards that may be unrealistic for you.

PATIENT: That 8 hours of sleep is not necessarily a gold standard that applies to everyone and that even if on some days I am not fully rested, I may simply need to accept that and not jump to the conclusion that I slept poorly the night before and that I won't be able to function the next day.

THERAPIST: Very good! This should reduce your anxiety about sleep as well.

As shown in this scenario, some people with insomnia entertain unrealistic expectations about their sleep requirements and their daytime energy level. An important goal of cognitive therapy is to make those patients realize that diminished sleep and daytime energy are not always pathological, and that even good sleepers do not always obtain 8 hours of sleep and do not feel completely refreshed every morning. Those individuals may benefit from reappraising their expectations.

Vignette 2

In the second scenario, the therapist is attempting to reappraise and decatastrophize the perceived impact of insomnia on daytime functioning and health.

> "After a poor night's sleep, I know that it will interfere with my daily activities the next day."
> "I am concerned that chronic insomnia may have serious consequences on my health."

THERAPIST: You believe quite strongly that you won't be able to function during the day after a poor night's sleep and that you might eventually get sick because of insomnia. Is that right?

PATIENT: Yes, it is.

THERAPIST: Let's take a closer look at the first concern that you're not able to function during the day after a poor night's sleep. Have there been times when this has happened?

PATIENT: Of course, there have!

THERAPIST: Would you say that every time you had a poor night's sleep you were unable to function the next day?

PATIENT: Well, maybe not every time.

THERAPIST: Can you remember times when you were able to function fairly well during the day despite having slept poorly the preceding night?

PATIENT: Euh... yes! I guess it has happened.

THERAPIST: Conversely, have there been times when you had difficulties functioning or had no energy during the day even after a good night's sleep?

PATIENT: Yes, that has happened several times as well.

THERAPIST: So, it sounds like your appraisal is not entirely accurate and that your level of functioning is not totally dependent on the quality of your sleep. Would you agree with that assessment?

PATIENT: Yes. I have never realized that before.

THERAPIST: Is it also possible that you worry about other things in life that may also interfere with your daytime functioning or with your energy level?

PATIENT: This is quite possible. In fact, I have been worrying quite a bit lately about my mother's health; she has just undergone surgery for breast cancer. I guess this has been worrying me a great deal more than I realized.

THERAPIST: So, would it be fair to say that this worrying alone could also take some of your energy and interfere with your ability to function during the day.

PATIENT: I guess so. You're right.

THERAPIST: Now, how could we reformulate this belief in a more realistic way?

PATIENT: Well that could be something like: "Insomnia is not the only cause of poor functioning during the day. Also, even if I feel more tired during the day after a poor night's sleep, most of the time I can still function pretty good".

THERAPIST: Very good! And you might even add that the more you worry about those daytime impairments, the greater the chance it will affect your sleep the next night. This is like a self-fulfilling prophecy. . . . Now, let's take a look at the other concern that you could get sick because of insomnia. Have you ever heard that someone died because of insomnia?

PATIENT: (Smile). No, I haven't.

THERAPIST: Would you say that poor sleepers are all sicker than good sleepers?

PATIENT: Probably not. I know good sleepers who are sicker than me.

THERAPIST: It is clear that insomnia causes fatigue and may make you feel bad the next day, but there is no evidence that it is necessarily detrimental to your health. So, again, what alternative, more realistic, thoughts can we identify?

PATIENT: Hmm . . . Something like: "Insomnia may be very unpleasant but it is not dangerous to my health"

THERAPIST: Excellent! How about adding this one: "Excessive worrying about insomnia may be more detrimental to health than sleep loss itself".

PATIENT: Yes that's probably right as well!

There is a tendency among insomnia sufferers to amplify the consequences of sleep disturbances. Because they can become quite obsessed by those potential consequences, some individuals are not even aware of this tendency. Providing accurate information about the objective consequences of insomnia is often very reassuring. Sometimes, it is necessary to use more directive methods to bring the patient to see that his or her subjective complaints about daytime impairments are magnified and disproportionate in relation to objective deficits. A verbal intervention such as the "Descending Arrow Technique" can be particularly helpful to decatastrophize insomnia. The therapist simply ask the patient "What is the worst that could happen if you did not sleep tonight", and the next worst scenario, etc. Such intervention can bring some relief and reduce the fear of insomnia.

Vignette 3

The third example illustrates the use of reattribution techniques to modify some misconceptions about the causes of insomnia.

"I feel insomnia is basically the result of a chemical imbalance"
"I feel I have very little control over my sleep"

THERAPIST: People often have their own idea about what is causing their sleep problem. You seem to agree fairly strongly with the belief that insomnia is the result of a chemical imbalance. What does that mean for you?

PATIENT: I have no idea what is causing my sleep problem but I am pretty sure there must be some chemical imbalance.

THERAPIST: And, if this were true, what would that mean to you?

PATIENT: This means that I can't do anything about it, that nobody can help me, that I am helpless.

THERAPIST: And how does that make you feel.

PATIENT: I am very distressed about this and about the whole idea that I may have to live with insomnia the rest of my life.

THERAPIST: Is it possible that other factors might be involved as well?

PATIENT: I guess so, but I have no idea what they are.

THERAPIST: What factors do you think might cause insomnia in other people?

PATIENT: I'm sure stress and anxiety play a big role in sleep difficulties.

THERAPIST: You are right! These are some of the most common causes of insomnia. Can you think of any specific examples?

PATIENT: Well, I guess that after an argument with my spouse, I tend to worry about it when I get to bed and it disrupts my sleep.

THERAPIST: So, this would also apply to your own experience?

PATIENT: Yes, it would.

THERAPIST: Can you think of another example?

PATIENT: Well, if I fall asleep involuntarily while watching television in the evening, I know it will take longer to fall asleep when I go to bed later that evening.

THERAPIST: This is a very good example. Is it also possible that when you worry about not sleeping and about how it will affect you the next day, it may aggravate your sleep problem.

PATIENT: I think you are right but I don't always realize that I worry about sleep.

THERAPIST: Now, can you think of any event or activities that might help you sleep better at night.

PATIENT: I know that when I have been fairly active during the day and have enjoyed a relaxed evening, I tend to sleep better at night.

THERAPIST: Good! So, it sounds like there are several factors other than a chemical imbalance that may actually affect your sleep.

PATIENT: I guess so.

THERAPIST: Does that mean that something can be done to improve your sleep?

PATIENT: I guess so too.

THERAPIST: So, how could we change your belief that "My insomnia is essentially the result of a chemical imbalance"?

PATIENT: Well, I could say that there is never just one cause to insomnia. . . .

THERAPIST: Exactly!. . . . And you could add that you do have some control in changing some of those causes.

PATIENT: Yes, you're right.

THERAPIST: Great! How do you feel about that now?

PATIENT: I feel less distressed about the whole thing and a bit more confident that I can do something to improve my condition. May be I am not so helpless after all.

As shown in this example, some individuals tend to attribute their insomnia solely to external factors (e.g., chemical imbalance, pain, aging); such external attributions are often accompanied by the underlying belief that nothing can be done to overcome insomnia. That is, because of this chemical imbalance one is condemned to suffer sleep disturbance indefinitely or else, drug is the only possible cure. It is critical to explain that insomnia is rarely caused by a single factor; it is often a multidimensional problem. As such, behavioral and psychological factors are always involved in maintaining insomnia, regardless of the primary etiological factors. The patient can then be encouraged to change some of those factors he or she has some control over (e.g., reducing time spent in bed; avoiding naps).

TREATMENT IMPLEMENTATION ISSUES

As may be obvious by now, cognitive therapy is essentially a verbal intervention that requires a great deal of convincing and persuasion. Some patients will respond to simple information and education, but others will require more systematic efforts to change their beliefs system.

Implementation of cognitive therapy is more time-consuming and requires more training for the clinician. As such, it may not be possible or desirable for all clinicians to implement this treatment component. The level of cognitive therapy that can be implemented will also vary with patients as a function of their educational level and psychological mindedness.

Very few patients present dysfunctional cognitions in every domains described earlier (i.e., sleep expectations, causal attributions). Conversely, there is always some dysfunctional sleep cognitions, even among those who fail to recognize such contributing factors. The clinician needs to adopt a detective-like attitude to uncover those cognitions and identify those domains that are most relevant for each patient.

It is important to implement cognitive therapy in appropriate dosage and timing. Because of the verbal nature of this intervention, it is best to spend no more than 15–20 minutes within a single consultation session to work on this therapeutic component. This amount of time is generally sufficient to communicate the main messages while retaining the patient's attention. It is also necessary to return to this treatment component during the course of several consecutive sessions. While cognitive therapy is usually best introduced after the behavioral therapy component, for some patients it may be necessary to work on those issues before attempting to implement behavioral procedures. Regardless of when cognitive therapy is introduced, the patient should complete the DBAS as part of the initial evaluation and keep a self-monitoring form of thoughts about sleep from baseline throughout the course of treatment.

When conducting cognitive therapy, both the source of the message must be credible and the content of the message must be conveyed with an appropriate tone. It is particularly important to avoid antagonizing the patient with statements such as "you are definitely getting more sleep than you think" or "insomnia has no consequence on daytime functioning and just stop worrying about it". Such statements are counterproductive and most likely would drive your patient away. The clinician must remain empathic and, at the same time, skillfully implement cognitive restructuring techniques to alter those misconceptions about sleep and insomnia.

Sometimes, patients may seem to agree with your verbal interventions but they may simply be reluctant to question the validity of your interventions and interpretations. It is essential to check with them if they understand what you are telling them, if it makes sense to them, and if it applies or not to their particular circumstances. Never take for granted that patients understand, accept, and integrate your argumentation. It is essential to validate the impact of your verbal interventions.

SUPPORTING EVIDENCE

Cognitive therapy has become an integral component of most multi-faceted treatment protocols for insomnia (Espie, Inglis, et al., 2001; Edinger, Wohlgemuth, Radtke, Marsh, Quilliam, 2001b; Morin, Colecchi et al. 1999). The nature of those interventions may range from formal cognitive restructuring therapy to psychoeducational intervention about age-appropriate sleep expectations/norms. Because cognitive therapy is typically combined with behavioral or educational interventions, it is not possible to determine its specific contribution to the overall outcome. Nonetheless, clinical evidence suggests that cognitive therapy is particularly useful to distinguish normal, age-related sleep changes, from pathological insomnia, and to reduce the emotional distress that is almost always associated with insomnia. Cognitive therapy is also instrumental to facilitate hypnotic discontinuation by reducing excessive apprehensions about withdrawal symptoms. The benefits of cognitive therapy extend beyond its initial impact on sleep parameters; some preliminary evidence suggests that this treatment modality may play an important function in mediating and maintaining long-term therapeutic outcome (Morin et al., 2002).

OTHER COGNITIVE APPROACHES

Several other cognitively-based intervention strategies may be effective in treating insomnia. We will present each of these fairly briefly.

Paradoxical Intention

We referred to the use of paradox earlier in this chapter. The proposition underlying this approach is that anxiety responses may be conditioned not only to external cues but also to the individual's own behavior (Ascher & Turner, 1979; Espie & Lindsay, 1985; Espie, 1991). Fear of a performance failure (insomnia) and of anticipated negative consequences of that failure is described as performance anxiety. In paradoxical treatment, counter-productive attempts to fall asleep are replaced by the intention of remaining passively awake or by giving up any direct effort to fall asleep. This rationale is supportable in that good sleepers do not use any strategies to fall asleep. Indeed effort to sleep may readily inhibit the natural sleep process (Espie, 2002). Evidence of this type of mechanism was provided also by Ansfield Wegner, and Bowser (1996) who reported paradoxical wakefulness among those attempting to sleep in circumstances of high mental load (e.g. stress), and by Harvey (in press) who found that subjects asked to suppress dominant thoughts while in bed were less successful at sleeping. Paradoxical intention has demonstrated efficacy in controlled trials (Turner & Ascher, 1979; Espie, Lindsay, Brooks, Hood, & Turvey, 1989) and is an intervention which reflects a 'moderate degree of clinical effectiveness' (Chesson et al., 1999).

You might consider offering your patients the following rationale and instructions.

> *If you can't get to sleep it might seem reasonable to ask someone who is a good sleeper how he/she manages it. What do you think they would say? Something like "I just fall asleep . . . it just happens . . . I don't do anything really?" You might think this is not very helpful, but the secret is right there—they do precisely nothing!*
>
> *Sleep is a natural process which happens involuntarily. The good sleeper doesn't make it happen, or have some kind of method that you don't know about it. You are the one with all the methods and tactics, and none of them works! To become a good sleeper you need to learn to abandon all your efforts to sleep because they simply get in the way of the natural process. They make you too self-conscious about your sleep and about your sleep failures. You know how sometimes you lie awake for ages or toss and turn until it's getting close to morning time? And you feel some relief as you think that soon you can get up? Why do you sometimes fall asleep at that point? That's because you give up trying then and you give up being concerned. How about having that as a general approach. Try this:*
>
> 1. *When you are in bed lie in a comfortable position and put the light out.*
> 2. *In the darkened room, keep your eyes open, and try to keep them open "just for a little while longer." That's your catch phrase.*
> 3. *As time goes by, congratulate yourself on staying awake but relaxed.*
> 4. *Remind yourself not to try to sleep but to let sleep overtake you, as you gently try to resist it.*
> 5. *Keep this mind-set going as long as you can, and if you get worried at staying awake remind yourself that that is the general idea, so you are succeeding.*
> 6. *Don't actively prevent sleep by trying to rouse yourself. Be like the good sleeper; let sleep come to you.*

Many of your patients will identify with the fact that trying to sleep is self-defeating. In some ways insomnia can be seen as a disorder of sleep preoccupation. Paradoxical intention helps to overcome this preoccupation by encouraging the development of a more philosophical attitude toward wakefulness. We have recently developed an instrument called the Glasgow Sleep Effort Scale that you may find helpful in assessing sleep-related performance effort. This is reproduced in Appendix Q. This scale is useful as an assessment of the likely benefit of a paradoxical approach. By discussing ratings made on each item you will also be able to explain the rationale of this approach, an important matter if your patient is going to implement paradoxical intention correctly. If your patient has difficulty understanding the nature of paradox try helping them to stand back a bit from insomnia by considering other natural functions that can be impaired by preoccupation and by trying too much, such as stammering, erectile impotence and blushing.

Cognitive Control

This is a technique that we first described some years ago (Espie & Lindsay, 1987). It is really an extension of the idea of stimulus control, but recognizes that it is primarily thoughts and worries that seem to be incompatible with successful sleep. The great majority of people with insomnia report mental overarousal in bed. They complain of difficulty in emptying their minds and of racing thoughts. Cognitive control comprises a simple set of procedures to remove mental activity from the bed and bedroom environment, or at least to reduce the influence of cognitive activity upon sleep. These are the instructions that you would give to your patient.

Putting the day to rest.
You may find this technique particularly useful for thoughts that have to do with the past day and planning for the following day. The aim is to put the day to bed, along with your plans for the next day . . . so that you can get to sleep". If you can manage to stop the thinking you usually do in bed, before it happens, then you should sleep better.
*   To put the day to rest:*
1. Set aside 20 minutes in the early evening (say around 7 p.m.) and sit down with a pen and a notebook.
2. Think of what has happened during the day, how it has gone, and how you feel about it—evaluate things.
3. Write down anything you need to do on a 'to do' list, and any steps that you can take to complete any loose ends.
4. Try to use your 20 minutes to leave you feeling more organized and in control and close the notebook when you are done.
5. When it comes to bedtime remind yourself that you have already dealt with things when they come to your mind.
6. If new thoughts come up note them down on a piece of paper at your bedside, to be dealt with the next day.

Cognitive control is like a pre-emptive strike upon insomnia! Intrusive and repetitive thoughts maintain arousal and disrupt sleep. If you can encourage your patients to prepare for bed in this way they are likely to benefit. Besides, it is not in itself dysfunctional to reflect and to plan. It is more a matter of when to do it! You may find it helpful to incorporate cognitive control along with the 'bedtime wind down' procedures described in Chapter 4 and the section on 'making the connection between bed and sleep' presented in Chapter 5 as part of the stimulus control procedure.

Thought-Blocking

A final cognitive technique worth mentioning is thought-blocking. This has obvious appeal, again because of the disruptive nature of pre-sleep mentation. However, people usually say that they have tried to block out thoughts . . . but unsuccessfully. They may in fact complain that trying to do so makes them worse. This may seem unsurprising now that we have discussed the paradoxical nature of sleep. Indeed, there is some evidence that thought suppression may be a counterproductive strategy employed by poor sleepers (Harvey, in press).

Rather than actively trying to suppress thoughts and thought content, we suggest that, where the mental material is predictable, such as rehearsing the day that is past and planning for tomorrow, you instruct your patient in the cognitive control procedures above. Likewise, you might suggest relaxation with imagery training (see Chapter 4) when the intrusive thought content is "flighty," jumping from topic to topic, because imagery may help sustain a more relaxed mental theme. However, there is one technique, that is a form of thought-blocking, that we can recommend.

"Articulatory suppression" is a technique widely used in studies of working memory. The phonological component of the central executive is referred to as the articulatory loop, which serves to hold in store the verbal elements required in any cognitive task. Levey, Aldaz, Watts, & Coyle (1991) applied articulatory suppression techniques to the treatment of insomnia. They thought that, by blocking up this short-term store with semantically meaningless phonemes, no other mental information would be processed. They presented an interesting case series supporting this contention, particularly for sleep maintenance insomnia i.e. using the technique at any wakening from sleep.

Here are the instructions for articulatory suppression to give to patients:

1. *While lying in bed with your eyes closed*
2. *Repeat the word "the" once or twice every second in your head*
3. *Don't say it out loud, but it may help if you "mouth it"*
4. *Keep up these repetitions for about 5 minutes or until sleep ensues*

You should also provide a simplified version of the above rationale to your patient. One way of doing this is to explain a little about the workings of short-term memory e.g. how it is that we need to rehearse even just a few digits (like in an unknown telephone number) if we are to remember it at all. You can further explain that during that rehearsal time we cannot allow anything else into our mind because it will erase the brief memory. So it is also the other way round that if we have something meaningless occupying that space in our thinking processes nothing much else can squeeze past. A recent study by Harvey and Payne (2002) also showed that an imagery distraction procedure was useful in the management of unwanted pre-sleep thoughts in insomnia.

These additional cognitive techniques of paradoxical intention, cognitive control and articulatory suppression can be used to complement formal cognitive therapy, and as an adjunct to the more behaviorally-based interventions presented in the preceding chapters.

Sleep Medications

INTRODUCTION

Two different scenarios regarding sleep medications are likely to arise in the clinical management of insomnia. The first one involves patients who do not use medication and are reluctant to do so, although they might benefit from an occasional sleep aid. The second one, most commonly encountered by psychologists, involves patients who have already been on medications for a prolonged period but, despite several attempts, have been unable to discontinue their use. In this chapter, we address the management of insomnia in both of these scenarios. In the first section, we present an overview of medications available for treating insomnia, with a summary of their benefits, risks and limitations, their indications and contra-indications, and clinical guidelines on their appropriate use. The second part presents a step-by-step protocol to facilitate hypnotic discontinuation among prolonged users.

TYPES OF MEDICATIONS USED FOR INSOMNIA

Several classes of medications are used in the treatment of insomnia. They include the traditional benzodiazepines (BZD), non-benzodiazepine hypnotics, antidepressants, antihistamines, and several herbal and dietary supplements available without prescriptions.

Benzodiazepine-Receptor Agents

There are several BZDs that are specifically marketed as hypnotics (e.g., temazepam, nitrazepam) and several more (e.g., lorazepam,

Table 7.1. Benzodiazepine-Receptor Agents Commonly Prescribed for Insomnia

Benzodiazepines	Equivalent dosage (mg)[a]	Usual dosage (mg)	Half-life[b] (hours)
Bromazepam[c] (Lectopam®)	3	1.5–6	8–19
Clonazepam (Klonopin®)	0.25	0.5–2	20–60
Estazolam (ProSom®)	1	1.0–2.0	8–24
Flurazepam (Dalmane®)	15	15–30	48–100
Lorazepam (Ativan®)	1	0.5–2	10–20
Nitrazepam[c] (Mogadon®)	10	5–10	16–18
Oxazepam (Serax®)	15	10–30	5–10
Temazepam (Restoril®)	15	7.5–30	8–17
Triazolam (Halcion®)	0.25	0.125–0.25	2–4
Quazepam (Doral®)	15	7.5–30	40–120
Zaleplon (Sonata®)	5	5–10	1
Zopiclone[c] (Imovane®)	3.75	3.75–7.5	4–6
Zolpidem (Ambien®, Stilnox®)	5	5–10	1.5–5

[a] A dosage of 1 mg of lorazepam is equivalent to 15 mg of temazepam.
[b] May be longer in older adults.
[c] Not available in the United State The commercial name of some drugs may vary across countries.

oxazepam) which, although marketed as anxiolytics, are frequently used for insomnia as well. In addition, there are three newer hypnotics (zolpidem, zopiclone, and zaleplon), which are not benzodiazepines per se, but they act on the same benzodiazepine and gamma aminobutyric acid-a receptors ($GABA_A$). Unlike the traditional BZDs, which all have hypnotic, anxiolytic, and anticonvulsant properties, these newer drugs have more selective hypnotic effects. Table 7.1 presents a list of those medications commonly used in the pharmacological treatment of insomnia, and which are often grouped together under benzodiazepines receptor agonists (BRAs). This class of medications presents a lower risk of physical dependence and lethal overdose compared to older drugs such as chloral hydrate and the barbiturates (American Psychiatric Association, 1990; Roy-Byrne & Cowley, 1991). Their therapeutic and side effect profiles are comparable, although medications with rapid onset and short-to-intermediate duration of action have the best ratio of benefits to residual effects. Their main difference is in their pharmacokinetic properties: absorption, distribution, and elimination. Combined with the dosage, these properties mediate the effects of the drugs on sleep and on daytime functioning (Greenblatt, 1991; Roehrs & Roth, 2000). We will return to those effects after a brief overview of other drugs used for insomnia.

Antidepressants

Antidepressants with sedating properties are often used in the treatment of insomnia, alone or in combination with hypnotics (Buysse & Reynolds, 2000). Those antidepressants most commonly used include trazodone, amitriptyline, trimipramine, and doxepin. These agents are used in smaller doses for treating insomnia (e.g., 10–20 mg of amitriptyline) than they are for treating depression. Trazodone is fairly sedating and improves sleep continuity and increases slow-wave sleep. Tricyclics such as amitriptyline and doxepin may also improve sleep continuity but they produce a significant reduction of REM sleep. The newer generations of antidepressants, the selective serotonin reuptake inhibitors (SSRI), such as fluoxetine and sertraline, are generally more stimulating and may actually produce insomnia when used at bedtime. Some antidepressants (tricyclics, fluoxetine) may also exacerbate periodic limb movements during sleep. Although antidepressants with sedating properties can be very helpful for the management of sleep disturbances among depressed patients, very few studies have examined the efficacy and safety of those agents when used as hypnotics with non-depressed insomniacs (e.g., Hohagen et al., 1994). Therefore, antidepressants are not recommended as the first line of treatment for primary insomnia.

Antihistamines

The active ingredient in most of the widely available over-the-counter preparations for insomnia (e.g., Sominex, Nytol, Sleep-Eze, Unisom) is an antihistamine such as diphenhydramine or doxylamine. Those agents produce drowsiness and, despite their widespread use as sleep aids, very few studies have evaluated the efficacy and safety of antihistamines as hypnotics (Rickels et al., 1983). The evidence suggests that diphenhydramine may be useful for mild insomnia, but there is no evidence that it is efficacious in the treatment of chronic and severe insomnia. In addition, antihistamines can produce adverse (psychomotor and cognitive impairments) and residual effects the next day (e.g., sleepiness). Some patients may also report a paradoxical effect (i.e., agitation rather than drowsiness).

Herbal and Dietary Supplements

Melatonin is another agent that is frequently used as a sleep aid. It is a naturally occurring hormone produced by the pineal gland at night. It may be useful for some forms of circadian sleep disturbances associated with shift-work and jet-lag, but its benefits for insomnia are equivocal and the adverse effects with long-term usage are unknown (Mendelson, 1997). Although it is widely available in over-the-counter preparations, the use of melatonin for insomnia is premature at this time. Several herbal products (e.g., valerian, chamomile, kava) are increasingly used as sleep aid. Of those, valerian extracts are among the most widely used herbal remedies for insomnia. Evidence from clinical studies indicate modest sedative and anxiolytic effects and few residual effects (Stevenson & Ernst, 2000). Despite their increasing popularity and widespread use, controlled studies are needed to evaluate further the risks and benefits of dietary and herbal products for sleep. As those products are not regulated by FDA, a major concern is that there is no guarantee for the consumers that the substances used in the various preparations correspond to the product labels.

CLINICAL BENEFITS, RISKS, AND LIMITATIONS

The evidence from controlled clinical trials indicates that benzodiazepine-receptor agents are effective in the acute and short-term management of insomnia (Holbrook, Crowther, Lotter, Cheng & King, 2000; Nowell et al., 1997; Parrino & Terzano, 1996; Smith et al., 2002). Those medications improve sleep continuity and efficiency through a reduction of sleep onset latency and time awake after sleep onset. They also reduce the number of awakenings and stage shifts through the night. Total sleep time is increased by an average of 45 to 60 minutes. Their effects on sleep stages vary with the specific class of medications. All BRAs increase stage 1 and stage 2 sleep. Benzodiazepines reduce slow-wave (stages 3–4) sleep and, to a lesser extent, REM sleep. Although stages 3–4 sleep are considered the deepest and most restorative sleep, the clinical significance of these alterations is unclear. These changes are less pronounced with the newer agents such as zolpidem, zopiclone, and zaleplon (Wagner, Wagner, & Hening, 1998). Overall, the evidence is fairly clear that hypnotic medications are efficacious for the acute and short-term treatment of insomnia.

However, clinical trials have generally been conducted over a 4 to 6 week period, and there are no controlled studies of their long-term efficacy.

The main limitations of hypnotic medications are their residual effects the next day and their associated risks of tolerance and dependence. The most common residual effects include daytime drowsiness, dizziness or lightheadedness, and impairments of cognitive and psychomotor functions. In general, side effects are minor and infrequent when medication is used at the appropriate dose, although there are always patients who cannot tolerate medications, hypnotics or others. Also, long-acting agents (e.g., flurazepam) are more likely to produce residual effects the next day (e.g., drowsiness). On the other hand, benzodiazepines can produce antero-grade amnesia, a problem that is more likely with shorter acting agents. With regular and prolonged usage, there is a risk of tolerance so that it may be necessary to increase the dosage to maintain therapeutic effects. Tolerance varies across agents and individuals, and some people may remain on the same dosage for prolonged periods of time. Whether this prolonged usage is a sign of continued effectiveness or of fear of discontinuing the medication is unclear. "Rebound insomnia" is a common problem associated with discontinuation of hypnotics; it is more pronounced with short-acting drugs and can be attenuated with a gradual tapering regimen (Gillin, Spinweber, & Johnson, 1989; Soldatos, Dikeos & Whitehead, 1999). Zolpidem and zopiclone may produce less rebound insomnia upon discontinuation, but patient's apprehension can exacerbate sleep disturbances upon discontinuation of any agent that was perceived to alleviate insomnia. Finally, all sleep-promoting medications, prescribed or over-the-counter, carry some risk of dependence (APA, 1990), which is often more psychological than physical. We will return to this topic in the second part of this chapter.

INDICATIONS AND CONTRAINDICATIONS

The main indication for hypnotic medications is situational insomnia, usually arising from acute stress, medical illness or hospitalization, and changes in the sleep environment or sleep schedules (jet lag, shift work). For persistent insomnia, a short-term trial of sleep medications may be indicated during the initial intervention in order to break the cycle of sleeplessness and emotional distress. For individuals who are not responsive to CBT, medications may be a useful alternative. Sleep medications may also be a useful adjunct for insomnia secondary to psychopathology (e.g., generalized anxiety disorders), although the main focus of treatment should be on the underlying condition. It may also be useful in the management of insomnia associated with a medical condition (e.g., pain) or with another sleep disorder (e.g., restless legs/periodic limb movements).

Hypnotic medications are generally contraindicated among patients who are abusing alcohol or drugs, patients with severe sleep apnea, pregnant women, among individuals who are on call (e.g., nurses, fireman) and may need to awake rapidly and go to work during their usual sleep period. With the latter group, hypnotics would then interfere with alertness and cognitive functions. Use of sleep medications should be monitored carefully among older adults (National Institutes of Health; NIH, 1991) and patients with hepatic, renal, or pulmonary diseases and among patients with severe psychiatric conditions such as psychoses and borderline personality disorders (Buysse & Reynolds, 2000; Roehrs & Roth, 2000; Stepanski, Zorich, & Roth, 1991).

CLINICAL GUIDELINES ON THE APPROPRIATE USE OF SLEEP MEDICATION

Most sleep experts agree that, when medication is indicated for primary insomnia, a benzodiazepine-receptor agent (i.e., benzodiazepines, zopiclone, zaleplon, and zolpidem) should be the first line of treatment. Selection of a specific hypnotic is based on several factors, including the type of insomnia (sleep onset vs. maintenance difficulties), the individual's age, and the presence of comorbid medical or psychological conditions. The best hypnotic promotes sleep at night and leaves no or minimal residual effects the next day. As such, speed of onset of action and duration of effects are two important considerations in selecting a medication. Drugs with a rapid absorption rate and a short half-life (e.g., zolpidem, zaleplon) are better for sleep-onset insomnia, and those with an intermediate half-life (e.g., temazepam, lorazepam, zopiclone) are preferable for sleep-maintenance problems.

A general principle that applies to all sleep medications is to use the lowest effective dosage for the shortest period of time. Recommended dosages for the various drugs are provided in Table 7.1. It is best to start with the smallest dosage and to increase it only if necessary. Higher dosages will prolong the duration of action but they are also more likely to produce adverse effects the next day. Another standard recommendation is to use medication only as needed, about three times per week, and for no more than one month. Such guidelines may be adequate for acute and situational insomnia, but they are not realistic for several clinical situations that may require longer treatment.

Although intermittent usage may prevent tolerance, it may also promote dependency through a negative conditioning process. For example, after being awake for more than an hour (an aversive stimulus), the individual who takes a sleeping pill only occasionally is likely to get quick relief from sleeplessness. As such the "pill taking behavior" is negatively reinforced and is likely to re-occur in the near future. For this reason, some authors (Stepanski et al., 1991) have suggested to use sleep medications, not on a *prn* basis, but rather every night, over a limited period time, in order to avoid reinforcing this conditioning between sleeplessness and the "pill taking behavior". For the same reason, it may be preferable to use medication at a predetermined time (i.e., bedtime) rather than waiting an hour or two of wakefulness to get back up to take the medication.

Duration of treatment is also dependent on the course of insomnia. For acute insomnia, medications may be used for several consecutive nights. Ideally, treatment duration should not exceed a few nights in order to avoid tolerance and minimize the risk of dependency. If insomnia is a recurring problem and is predictable (e.g., when travelling), it may be necessary to repeat this treatment regimen periodically. For persistent insomnia, sleep medications may be used for up to 2–3 weeks to break the cycle of performance anxiety, but the main focus of therapy should be on behavioral and cognitive changes. When insomnia is a recurrent problem, it may be necessary to use medication on an intermittent basis.

Recent studies using an intermittent use, non-nightly, paradigm have shown that this method is as effective as a nightly use and is more acceptable to patients. In this paradigm, patients are instructed to take medication only on those nights when insomnia is expected or when performance is particularly important the next day (Hajak, 2002). The main advantages of this regimen is that patients, particularly those who do not experience insomnia every nights, would not need to use their medication every night. This regimen would then reduce the apprehension of becoming dependent with nightly use and give the patient a greater sense of being in control of treatment. This would also minimize tolerance and provide an alternative to those who may require long-term treatment. The main shortcoming of this paradigm is that sleep is often unpredictable among insomniacs, making it difficult to determine ahead of time when to use medication. There is also evidence that, in practice, patients tend to take sleep medication on a nightly or near nightly basis.

In summary, hypnotic medications are effective for the acute and short-term management of insomnia; they produce quick relief upon the very first night of usage and these benefits last several nights and, in some cases, up to a few weeks. There is currently little evidence of sustained benefits upon drug discontinuation or of continued efficacy with nightly and prolonged usage. In addition, all hypnotics carry some risk of dependence, particularly with prolonged usage. As several panels of insomnia experts have already concluded, the primary indication for hypnotic medications is for situational sleep difficulties; their role in the clinical management of persistent insomnia should be as an adjunct to behavioral interventions (NIH, 1984; 1991; 1996).

COMBINING PSYCHOLOGICAL AND PHARMACOLOGICAL APPROACHES

It is quite frequent in clinical practice that patients are first treated with medication by their primary care physician and, eventually, are referred to psychologists for behavioral treatment (Morin, 2001). Despite this common practice, is there evidence to support the combined treatment of insomnia? Theoretically, combining CBT and medication should optimize treatment outcome by capitalizing on the more rapid and potent effects of medication and the more sustained effects of cognitive-behavioral interventions. The limited evidence available, however, is not entirely clear as to whether a combined intervention has an additive or subtractive effect on long-term outcome. Only a handful of studies have evaluated the combined or differential effects of those treatment modalities. Three of those studies compared triazolam to relaxation (McClusky, Milby, Switzer, Williams, & Wooten, 1991; Milby et al., 1993) or sleep hygiene (Hauri, 1997), and the other one (Morin, Colecchi, Stone, Sood, & Brink, 1999) compared CBT to temazepam. Collectively, the evidence indicates that drug therapy produces quicker and slightly better results in the acute phase (first week) of treatment, whereas behavioral and drug therapies are equally effective in the short-term interval (4–8 weeks). Combined interventions have a slight advantage over single treatment modality during the initial course of treatment. Furthermore, sleep improvements are well sustained after behavioral treatment and those obtained with hypnotic drugs are quickly lost after discontinuation of the medication. Long-term outcome with combined therapies are more equivocal. Studies with short-term follow-ups (<1 month) indicate that a combined intervention (i.e., triazolam plus relaxation) produces more sustained benefits than drug therapy alone (McClusky et al., 1991; Milby et al., 1993), whereas the only two investigations with follow-ups exceeding six months in duration report more variable long-term outcomes among patients receiving a combined intervention relative to those treated with behavioral treatment alone (Hauri, 1997; Morin, Colecchi et al., 1999). It appears that some patients retain their initial sleep improvements whereas others return to their baseline values. Thus, despite the intuitive appeal in combining drug and non-drug interventions, it is not entirely clear where, how, and for whom it is indicated to combine behavioral and drug treatments for insomnia.

The few studies available on combined treatment have initiated and discontinued CBT and medication at the same time. To take full advantages of the quicker results from drug therapy and the more sustained effects of behavioral interventions, a sequential approach might be preferable to a combined (concurrent) approach. Recent studies in our laboratory (Vallières, 2002) have yielded promising results from a sequential approach, wherein medication was initiated first (either alone or in combination with CBT) and gradually discontinued and, most importantly, the behavioral intervention was continued after patients discontinued their medication. This sequential approach ensures that patients are still in treatment after drug tapering, hence providing an opportunity to integrate newly learned self-management skills, especially at a time when rebound insomnia is likely to reinforce the belief that medication is needed indefinitely.

In light of the important mediating role of psychological factors in persistent insomnia, behavioral and attitudinal changes are essential to sustain improvements in sleep patterns (Morin et al., 2002). When combining behavioral and drug therapies, there is always a chance that medication will undermine the patient's efforts in changing maladaptive behavioral patterns and dysfunctional cognitions. As such, patients' attributions of initial therapeutic benefits to the drug alone, without integration of self-management skills, may hinder long-term outcome and make the process of hypnotic discontinuation more difficult. Therefore, if your patient receives combined treatment, it is particularly important to provide some guidance to make sure that progress made in therapy is internalized and appropriately attributed to his efforts and behavioral changes rather than to the medication alone.

CLINICAL GUIDELINES FOR HYPNOTIC DISCONTINUATION

Although most individuals using sleep medications do so only for a limited period of time and have no trouble stopping it, some people use it for prolonged periods, often much longer than was intended initially. In this latter scenario, discontinuation of sleep medications often poses a significant challenge to clinicians and patients alike. This section presents clinical guidelines to facilitate discontinuation of hypnotic medications. After presenting a clinical vignette illustrating how people become dependent upon sleep medications, a conceptual model of hypnotic-dependent insomnia is presented and a step-by-step withdrawal protocol is outlined.

Susan is a 48 year-old woman, and mother of two teenagers, who has experienced insomnia ever since she separated from her husband more than 10 years ago. Her insomnia was initially associated with a great deal of stress surrounding the separation and a change of job occurring at about the same time. To help her get some sleep through this difficult period, her family doctor had prescribed 0.5 mg of lorazepam, to be used "only as needed". Initially, Susan was sleeping much better on those occasional nights she was using the medication. Before long, however, she was taking lorazepam several nights per week, mostly on weekdays, and eventually was using it even on weekends. Even after she had adjusted to the separation and to her new job, she continued using medication and started increasing the dosage to 1.0 mg, 1.5, and eventually 2 mg at bedtime. Although she did not like the idea of using sleep medication, whenever she attempted to stop it, it was only to find out that her sleep worsened. So, she was caught up in a vicious cycle of dependency on sleep medications.

The Natural History of Hypnotic-Dependent Insomnia

As this clinical vignette illustrates, sleep medication is typically initiated during periods of acute insomnia due to stress, medical illness or hospitalization, or simply when a person can no longer cope with the daytime sequelae of chronic sleep disturbance. Despite the initial intent to use medication only for a few nights, some people continue using it over a prolonged period because of persistent insomnia, but others may do so even after their sleep difficulties have subsided. For those latter people, sleep medications are used simply on a prophylactic basis, to prevent the recurrence of insomnia. The fear of not sleeping maintains the pill-taking behavior. With nightly use, tolerance may develop and increased dosage is sometimes necessary to maintain efficacy. When the maximum safe dosage is reached, the person is caught in a vicious cycle (see Figure 7.1). Although the medication may have lost its sleep-promoting effects, any attempt to stop it abruptly is followed by withdrawal symptoms and a worsening of sleep difficulties. This rebound insomnia, which is typically transient in nature (although it may last a few weeks in some cases), heightens the patient's anticipatory anxiety and reinforces the belief that he or she cannot sleep without medication. Naturally, this chain reaction is powerful in prompting the patient to resume usage of sleeping pill and, hence, the cycle of hypnotic-dependent insomnia.

Conditioning principles also play an important role in perpetuating drug use for insomnia. For example, the hypnotic (and anxiolytic) properties of most benzodiazepines alleviate an aversive state (i.e., sleeplessness); as such, the drug-taking behavior itself is negatively reinforced. Although

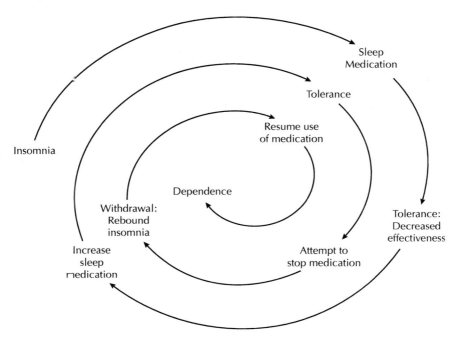

Figure 7.1 The cycle of hypnotic-dependent insomnia. *Source*: C.M. Morin (1993). *Insomnia: Psychological assessment and management*. New York: Guilford Press. Reproduced with permission.

sleeping pills are usually prescribed on an "as needed" basis in order to prevent tolerance, we have seen earlier in this chapter that such an intermittent schedule of administration can be quite powerful in perpetuating a habitual pattern of drug use. Another factor that may contribute to prolong hypnotic usage is the reversed sleep state misperception while under the influence of benzodiazepines. It is well recognized that unmedicated insomniacs overestimate the time required to fall asleep and underestimate total sleep time. Conversely, medicated insomniacs tend to have impaired recollection of wakefulness (i.e., they underestimate the amount of time spent awake) while on benzodiazepines and to perceive more sleep than is actually recorded by EEG measures. This phenomenon has been attributed to the amnesic properties of most benzodiazepines (Schneider-Helmert, 1988). Upon drug withdrawal, patients become acutely aware of their sleep disturbances, often prompting a quick return to drug use.

It is important to note that most prolonged users of sleep medications do not abuse their medications as some patients may abuse narcotics or stimulant drugs. Instead of escalating dosages beyond clinical recommendation, they simply continue using it longer than intended and are unable to stop it on their own. Nonetheless, this self-contained pattern of habitual and prolonged use will typically lead to dependency. Although this dependency has been documented primarily for benzodiazepines, it may also develop with other prescribed or even with over-the-counter sleep aids. As such, dependence upon sleep aids is often more psychological than physical in nature. The formal diagnosis of hypnotic-dependent insomnia involves a complaint of poor sleep with nearly daily use of a hypnotic agent for at least three weeks (ASDA, 1997). By definition, it also implies tolerance to hypnotics and withdrawal effects following discontinuation. This type of physical dependence is more likely to occur with high doses of benzodiazepines or with older hypnotic drugs (e.g., barbiturates). As most people remain on therapeutic doses without escalation for extensive periods of time, it is not entirely clear what proportion of long-term users meet criteria for hypnotic-dependent insomnia.

A Step-by-Step Approach to Discontinue Hypnotics

A step-by-step withdrawal protocol to discontinue hypnotic medications is described in this section. The procedures outlined here, or some variations of it, have been evaluated in several studies of benzodiazepines discontinuation with anxiety disorders patients and a few more with insomnia patients. The general principles of this medication tapering program can also be used with patients using other classes of medications (obtained with or without prescriptions) to promote sleep.

Evaluate patient's readiness and motivation. Before initiating drug tapering, it is essential to evaluate your patient's readiness and motivation about undertaking this program (Prochaska, DiClemente, & Norcross, 1992). If a person is still in a pre-contemplation phase (see Figure 5.2), it may not be indicated to initiate this program. It is also preferable to postpone it if the patient is under acute stress (e.g., recent death of a loved one). Tapering hypnotic drug is more likely to be successful if a patient's motivation is intrinsic (e.g., desire to achieve greater self-control) rather than extrinsic (e.g., pressure from a spouse). If the patient is reluctant to undertake a withdrawal program, it is important to determine whether lack of motivation or anticipatory anxiety is the main barrier. Providing information about the risks and adverse effects associated with use of sleeping pills may be a useful strategy initially but, ultimately, the patient should make the decision on his or her own. For patients who are apprehensive about withdrawal symptoms and rebound insomnia, simple information about the gradual tapering schedule and the transient nature of most withdrawal symptoms should alleviate those concerns. Other patients may have little self-confidence in their ability to discontinue medication; they should be encouraged to view this program as an opportunity to achieve greater self-control over their sleep and their life in general. You need to convey a high level of confidence about the process of discontinuation, but at the same time remain realistic about the outcome.

Select a target date. With your patient, set a date to begin the tapering program and a target date to be completely drug-free. The patient should let this date known to a spouse, relative, or to a good friend in order to build up his motivation and to obtain the needed support.

Self-monitoring and goal setting. Keeping a daily sleep/medication diary is an integral component of any insomnia treatment. Along with sleep parameters, your patient should keep a record of the type, frequency, and dosage of all sleep aids (prescribed or over-the-counter drugs, and alcohol). This may be achieved by incorporating nightly use of sleep medication and alcohol in the Sleep Diary (Chapter 3; Appendix B). Self-monitoring is completed for a 2-week baseline period and throughout treatment. In addition to establishing baseline, the diary is very helpful for monitoring progress, severity of symptoms, and compliance with the tapering regimen. Keep a summary log of the weekly amount of medication used and the number of medicated/drug-free nights (see Table 7.2).

A useful procedure to keep your patient focused and goal-oriented is to have him set a weekly goal for reductions in dosage and number of medicated nights. You might also ask your patients to indicate their self-efficacy level (% confidence) in achieving that goal. When this rating is too low, it may be necessary to keep the patient on the same schedule for an additional week in order to have him gain a greater sense of mastery before proceeding to a lower dosage. For example, if a patient is only 50% confident in reducing his lorazepam from 1.0 mg to 0.5 mg per night, this goal should be revised and made more attainable, or postponed until the next week. You can also enter weekly self-efficacy ratings on the form shown in Table 7.2.

Stabilization period. When two or more hypnotic drugs are used, either concomitantly or in alternance, you should first stabilize your patient on a single agent. For example, when a patient alternates between nitrazepam and triazolam, possibly to minimize tolerance, he should be stabilized on a single drug, in this case nitrazepam. When two benzodiazepines are used, it is preferable to retain the drug with the longer half-life because of its built-in tapering properties. Switching from a short- to a long-acting compound may minimize rebound effects. Table 7.1 provides information on equivalent benzodiazepine dosages. At the end of this stabilization

Table 7.2. A Sample Medication Withdrawal Schedule

Week	Type	Dosage (mg)	Number of nights	Total amount (mg)	% dosage reduction	Self-efficacy (0–100%)
Baseline	Lorazepam	2	7	14	—	—
Week 1	Lorazepam	1.5	7	10.5	25%	—
Week 2	Lorazepam	1.5	4	9	36%	—
		1.0	3			
Week 3	Lorazepam	1	7	7	50%	80%
Week 4	Lorazepam	1	4	5.5	61%	65%
		0.5	3			
Week 5	Lorazepam	0.5	7	3.5	75%	75%
Week 6	Lorazepam	0.5	5	2.5	82%	80%
Week 7	Lorazepam	0.5	5	2.5	82%	75%
Week 8	Lorazepam	0.5	3	1.5	89%	60%
Week 9	Lorazepam	0.5	1	0.5	96%	80%
Week 10	Lorazepam	0	0	0	100%	75%

period, which usually last 1–2 weeks, the patient should take only one drug at the same dosage every night and have ceased all other sleep aids, including alcohol and over-the-counter products.

Use a gradual tapering schedule. With regular and prolonged users of hypnotic medications, it is always preferable to follow a gradual withdrawal schedule rather than an abrupt discontinuation. This principle is intended to minimize withdrawal and rebound effects. The dosage is usually reduced by 25%, at intervals of 1–2 weeks, until the lowest available dosage is reached (see Table 7.2). For someone like Susan in our clinical vignette, the initial dosage of 2.0 mg of lorazepam was reduced to 1.5 mg, then to 1.0 mg, and to 0.5 mg. The total duration of the tapering program may vary between 4 and 12 weeks in outpatient settings, depending on the initial dosage, drug potency, and duration of use (DuPont, 1990; Lader, 1990; Rickels, Case, Schweizer, Garcia-Espana, & Fridman, 1990). In our experience, a period of 8–10 weeks has proved adequate for the large majority of patients using hypnotics at dosages that remained within therapeutic range (Baillargeon et al., in press; Morin, Colecchi, Ling, & Sood, 1995; Morin et al., 2003). This period may also vary as a function of withdrawal symptoms and patient's tolerance of those symptoms. When withdrawal symptoms are pronounced, it is best to slow the tapering schedule. Intervals of less than one week between dosage reduction are not recommended because of the associated risk of rebound insomnia, which can interfere with the tapering process and perpetuate the use of sleeping pills.

Introduce "drug holidays." Once the lowest available dosage is reached, it is time to introduce "drug holidays". Medication is allowed only on a number of predetermined nights. This will entail skipping one or two nights the first week, two or three nights the next week, and so on. The patient is asked to select in advance on which nights he/she will skip the sleeping pills. To minimize apprehension about impairments of day-time functioning, it is best to skip medication initially on nights when there are no major obligations the next day, usually on weekends. The next step is to schedule additional drug-free nights even when there is a full agenda on the next day. When medication intake is reduced to only a few nights per week, the patient is instructed to use it on a fixed schedule rather than on an as needed basis. As such, medication is used only on pre-selected nights (e.g., Sunday, Tuesday, and Thursday), and at a fixed time (i.e., 30 minutes before bedtime), independent of whether sleep difficulties are experienced or not. With this schedule, the patient is not allowed to use medication on some nights when he may, indeed, experience sleep difficulties. Conversely, he is obligated to use it on other nights when he might not need it. This "time-contingent" schedule is helpful to dissociate or weaken the association between sleeplessness and the drug-taking behavior.

Stop it! The final step is to stop completely the medication. This step is difficult for some patients who become anxious, or even obsessed, with the idea of giving up the last few micrograms of their pills and about the expected consequences it will have on their sleep. It may be reassuring to simply remind them that such a small quantity of medication may have very little therapeutic effect on sleep.

Relapse prevention. Of course, staying drug-free is often more difficult than the initial discontinuation. Patients may continue experiencing sleep difficulties for quite some time after hypnotic discontinuation, and remain vulnerable to resume medication. It is particularly important to inform them that it may take some time before sleep patterns return to normal. Patients should be guided to identify high-risk situations, both for insomnia and for use of sleeping pills (e.g., before an important deadline). Once those situations are identified, the patient may be in a better position to prevent major sleep difficulties (by restricting time in bed) or to cope with the occasional, but inevitable poor night's sleep. Cognitive therapy can be particularly useful to bring patients to see those occasional poor nights' sleep as resulting from identifiable causes (e.g., stress) rather than as evidence that persistent insomnia has returned. You should encourage your patient to develop greater tolerance to these occasional nights of poor sleep.

In spite of these measures, some patients will be unable to remain completely drug free. It is important to distinguish lapses from relapses and teach them not to catastrophize if they should have to use a sleep medication for one or two nights. On the other hand, they should also be encouraged to limit their usage to the occasional use of the smallest dosage available in order to avoid returning to the old pattern of drug-dependency. In order to prevent relapse and foster maintenance of therapeutic benefits, it may be necessary to plan a maintenance phase involving periodic phone calls or follow-up therapy sessions. You may find the motivation cycle diagram, presented in Chapter 5 (Figure 5.2), useful in helping patients to persist with their goal of becoming drug-free. For some patients, simply having a few hypnotics available at home to face an emergency situation may be enough to reduce anticipatory anxiety and actually prevent further insomnia and use of medications.

Clinical and Practical Issues

Withdrawal Implementation.   The majority of patients who are dependent on sleep medications can be managed on an outpatient basis. However, patients who are using more than twice the highest recommended dosages (e.g., 60 mg of flurazepam or temazepam) should be referred for inpatient detoxification. An inpatient program will provide a safer environment to reduce the medication and respond promptly to severe withdrawal symptoms (e.g., seizures). Whether implemented on an outpatient or inpatient setting, a physician should supervise/monitor the tapering program. A pharmacist may also play a very important role in designing the most appropriate tapering schedule.

Ideally, the patient should be seen once a week during the withdrawal period. During each of these visits, you should review the daily diary for hypnotic usage, withdrawal symptoms, and changes in sleep during the previous week. Then, you should agree upon objectives for the target dosage for the next week, and evaluate the patient's confidence level in achieving that goal. As previously mentioned, when the self-efficacy rating is too low, the weekly goal should be revised to be made more attainable.

Although brief weekly consultations of 15–20 minutes each may be adequate for implementing the medication tapering program alone, additional time is required when CBT is implemented concurrently. Whether or not formal psychological treatment is implemented, patients' apprehensions and unrealistic beliefs should be carefully examined and dealt with during consultations sessions. When patients display high levels of anxiety, it is helpful to give them the opportunity to call the clinician between scheduled visits. In our experience, patients seldom call, but they are reassured to have this opportunity available in case of an emergency. Sometimes, it is also helpful to give patients the permission to use a small extra dose if an emergency situation arise or withdrawal symptoms become too severe. To foster a sense of mastery, patients should be given as much control as possible over the implementation of their drug tapering regimen. They should be involved in deciding when to initiate the withdrawal program, by how much the medication should be reduced on any given week, and when to introduce nights without medication.

Practical problems may arise in cutting down medication when the lowest available dosage has been reached. For example, it may be difficult to cut in half the smallest available dose (0.5 mg) of lorazepam or to reduce by 25% a capsule of 15 mg of temazepam. Also, for older adults who may have more dexterity problems, a pill-cutter can be purchased at the pharmacy. A temazepam capsule could be dissolved in 100 ml of water or juice and the patient could drink the quantity corresponding to the desire dose (e.g. 75 ml if the desired reduction is 25% of 15 mg).

Withdrawal Symptoms. The most likely withdrawal symptoms associated with benzodiazepine discontinuation include insomnia, anxiety, restlessness, increased perceptual acuity, and impaired concentration. There is a great deal of variability in terms of who experiences those symptoms and to what exten (O'Common et al., 1999). It is sometimes difficult to distinguish between persisting withdrawal symptoms and re-emergence of pre-morbid insomnia and anxiety symptoms. Several drug- and patient-related factors influence their incidence and severity. Withdrawal symptoms are more frequent among younger patients, women, and patients under chronic stress and those with pre-existing anxiety, depression and dependent personality (Rickels, Case et al., 1990). The most important drug-related factors are dosage, half-life, and duration of use. Withdrawal symptoms are more severe and more immediate with higher dosages and with short half-life (e.g. triazolam) than with long acting (e.g. flurazepam) benzodiazepines (Busto et al., 1986; Schweizer, Rickels, Case & Greenblatt, 1990). More severe symptoms (e.g., seizures, persistent tinnitus) may follow abrupt discontinuation of high doses of benzodiazepines. Gradual withdrawal minimizes the occurrence of those symptoms. Finally, when treatment duration is less than 2 weeks there is minimal rebound insomnia upon hypnotic discontinuation; however, withdrawal symptoms are more likely after prolonged usage.

Drug Substitution. Drug substitution may be useful to minimize withdrawal symptoms among patients using high dosages of benzodiazepines. Substitution of a long-acting benzodiazepine (e.g., diazepam, clonazepam) for short-acting ones before initiating withdrawal may reduce/postpone withdrawal symptoms (Ashton, 1994; APA, 1990). After a stabilization period of 1–2 weeks, a gradual tapering of the long-half life benzodiazepine is done as described above. Long half-life benzodiazepines may facilitate the reduction of medication initially, but withdrawal symptoms are not completely eliminated with longer acting agents, they are simply delayed. It is also possible to switch from a benzodiazepine to one of the more recent agents such as zopiclone or zolpidem, which have more specific hypnotic actions without anxiolytic effects. Several other drugs (phenobarbital) have been used to facilitate benzodiazepine discontinuation among anxiety disorders patients and among hospitalized patients with mixed chemical dependency (benzodiazepine with alcohol or other drugs) (APA, 1990). Although such substitution may be useful for those special populations, the large majority of insomnia patients seen in clinical practice have developed a drug dependency that is more psychological than pharmacological in nature. For this reason, it is difficult to have those patients switch from one pill, of a particular shape and color, to another format. In our experience, attempts at substituting a long-acting for a short-acting benzodiazepine have not been successful. In most cases, it is simply easier to work with the medication the patient has been using for months or even years.

Concurrent Psychological Interventions. Although a systematic and supervised drug tapering program may be sufficient for some individuals, most long-term users will benefit from the addition of cognitive-behavioral therapy. CBT is likely to help patients cope with the sleep disturbances that may arise or worsen during the tapering period as well as with some of the other withdrawal symptoms (e.g., anxiety). The nature and extent of this concurrent intervention will vary according to the patient's needs and severity of withdrawal symptoms and sleep difficulties. For some, simple encouragement, support, and education about the transient nature of withdrawal symptoms and rebound effects may be sufficient to get them through the discontinuation process. Others who are anxious even before withdrawal will benefit from relaxation training. Patients engaged in maladaptive sleep habits and who endorse dysfunctional sleep cognitions may require formal cognitive-behavioral therapy. Sleep restriction can minimize rebound insomnia during the tapering period and cognitive therapy can help to guide patients in reappraising withdrawal symptoms as temporary and manageable. Paradoxical methods (see Chapter 6) may also be helpful in assisting your patient to accept their situation rather than engaging in vain efforts to sleep well.

A related issue that often arises in clinical practice is whether drug tapering should be implemented before, during, or after behavioral treatment for insomnia. We have previously compared two withdrawal protocols, one in which five chronic hypnotic users were withdrawn before and five after receiving behavioral therapies (i.e., relaxation training, stimulus control, and paradoxical intention) (Espie et al., 1988). Patients who were withdrawn from medication early in treatment achieved a better outcome on sleep-onset latency than those withdrawn after behavior therapy. Four patients (one in the early and three in the late withdrawal) had resumed usage of hypnotic medication at the 1-year follow-up. Thus, it may be preferable to initiate the medication tapering early on, although maintenance therapy in the form of periodic booster sessions or phone calls may be necessary to prevent relapse in the long-run.

Evidence for Efficacy of Hypnotic Discontinuation Programs

Several studies have examined the efficacy of different withdrawal protocols to assist patients in benzodiazepine discontinuation. The majority of those studies have been conducted with anxiety patients using benzodiazepines as anxiolytics (e.g., Fraser, Peterkin, Gamsu, & Baldwin, 1990; Otto et al., 1993), and a few more have focused on insomnia patients using either benzodiazepines or other agents as hypnotic medications (e.g., Baillargeon et al., in press; Espie, Lindsay, & Brooks, 1988; Kirmil-Gray, Eagleston, Thorensen, & Zarcone, 1985; Lichstein & Johnson, 1993; Lichstein, Peterson et al., 1999; Morin et al., 1995; Morin et al., 2003).

The evidence currently available indicates that a supervised taper combined with psychological treatment produce significant reduction in the quantity and frequency of hypnotic medications used by insomnia patients. Between 70% and 80% of long-term hypnotic users are drug-free after an average of 8 to 10 weeks. Although promising, these short-term benefits must be tempered against long-term outcomes, as significant relapse rates may occur at intermediate (6-month) and long-term (12-month) follow-ups. As for other forms of substance abuse/dependency, it seems essential to integrate formal relapse prevention training in order to maintain therapeutic gains. Indeed, we have found that 4 out of 5 relatively unselected, clinic-presenting patients on hypnotics remained drug-free at 12 months following a CBT course with support in tapering and withdrawal (Espie et al., 2001).

In terms of treatment modality, the evidence indicates that a supervised tapering regimen is an essential therapeutic component to discontinue benzodiazepines among older adults. Brief consultations integrated into a structured, time-limited, and gradual tapering regimen is very important in keeping patients focused and goal-oriented. On the other hand, behavioral treatment of insomnia, without specific guidance in reducing hypnotic medications, may not be sufficient for long-term users who may have failed several previous attempts to discontinue medications on their own. The addition of psychological treatment to drug tapering enhances therapeutic benefits; it facilitates benzodiazepine discontinuation and reduces withdrawal symptoms. In addition, CBT specifically targeting insomnia improves sleep more than discontinuation of hypnotic medications alone. Sleep improvements, although modest initially, become more noticeable after patients have been off medication for several weeks or months.

CONCLUSIONS

Medication is often part of the management of insomnia. There is little doubt that it can be useful in the short-term treatment of insomnia, but its role in the long-term management of insomnia is more controversial because of the lack of evidence base. Despite the risks of tolerance and dependence, some people continue using sleep medications much longer than was initially intended. This is illustrative of the considerable unmet need for insomnia care in the general community. The management of those patients can be a challenging task but current evidence indicates that a supervised medication tapering, alone or combined with formal CBT, can be very effective to guide them in discontinuing hypnotic medications. A structured medication taper may be sufficient for some patients but the addition of formal cognitive-behavior therapy, specifically targeting insomnia and withdrawal symptoms (e.g., anxiety), appear to facilitate drug discontinuation by minimizing sleep disruptions during the withdrawal program.

Clinical and Treatment Implementation Issues

INTRODUCTION

This concluding chapter addresses practical guidelines for optimal treatment implementation. We discuss the advantages and limitations of different models for implementing therapy and outline best treatment parameters in terms of duration, frequency, and timing of consultation sessions. Common obstacles arising during therapy and strategies to promote treatment compliance are described. We conclude with some comments about the treatment of insomnia in special populations such as older adults and patients presenting comorbid medical and psychological disorders.

TREATMENT IMPLEMENTATION FORMATS: INDIVIDUAL, GROUP, AND BRIEF CONSULTATION MODELS

The treatment program described in this manual can be implemented successfully on an individual basis or in a group format. Each format has its own advantages and limitations. The main advantage of individual therapy is that treatment can be tailored to the specific needs and particularities of each individual. For instance, relaxation may be very helpful for some individuals but may actually be counter-productive for others. Likewise, although we generally introduce behavioral procedures (e.g., sleep restriction and stimulus control) as the first therapy component, it may be more appropriate and even necessary for some individuals with obvious dysfunctional beliefs to implement cognitive therapy early on to address those faulty cognitions that might impede adherence with behavioral procedures. For example, a person who is convinced that insomnia is detrimental to health may not be willing to readily change some maladaptive coping strategies (spending excessive amounts of time in bed, napping) unless the underlying belief is also modified. Another advantage of individual therapy is the flexibility it provides to target clinical issues (e.g., family/marital problems) or co-existing dysfunctions (anxiety or depression) that may interfere with the therapeutic process and impede sleep improvements. The flexibility of individual therapy, however, may also increase the risk of slowing down the therapeutic process. If therapy becomes too flexible, there is always a risk to move on more tangential topics that may not be directly related to insomnia. As a result, you may find that even after 8–10 therapy sessions, the essentials of insomnia therapy have not yet been covered completely.

In addition to its cost-effectiveness, group therapy offers several advantages. First, the opportunity to share a sleep problem with others and to realize that one is not alone can be of great comfort. Second, the group forum also serves as a powerful social support network for the participants. Third, model patients who diligently adhere to treatment can prove strong therapist' allies. The group format may also have a social inhibition role and prevent some people from bringing up materials or personal problems that may not be directly relevant to sleep difficulties. What should be the ideal group size? Between 5 and 7 persons seems to be the optimal number of participants for this type of structured, sleep-focused, intervention. With this number, the therapist can still individualize his or her treatment recommendations to each participant. For example, the sleep window can be calculated based on each individual's sleep diary data. A group of this size is also less intimidating, both for participants and therapists, than one with 10–12 people; as such, it increases the chance that each individual will be involved in group discussions. It is also possible to run larger groups (>10 people) but these group sessions become more like lectures and there are generally fewer interactions among participants and with the clinician. With a larger group, it is also more difficult for the therapist to keep track of each participant's difficulties and to provide individual attention to address those difficulties during therapy.

It is not always desirable or possible to treat insomnia in a group format. To run a group effectively, there must be some homogeneity among group members, particularly in terms of primary and secondary diagnoses. It is easier to conduct group therapy with individuals who present primary insomnia. The presence of a co-existing medical or psychological problems does not necessarily preclude enrollment in group therapy, but enrollment of patients with a significant comorbid condition, particularly an Axis II (personality) disorder, is discouraged as it is very likely to interfere with the group process. Participants should also be informed that, even if the medium of therapy is a group format, therapy is very structured and sleep-focused. As such, they should not expect or have to share in great details their childhood or life experience during those sessions. On the practical side, insomnia group therapy is usually closed, so that all participants initiate and complete therapy at the same time. For this reason, it is necessary to have a sufficient number of people with insomnia at a given time to initiate a new group. This is easier done as part of a clinical research program than it is in a general clinical practice. Despite the apparently long waiting lists of patients with insomnia at some sleep clinics, the announcement of group therapy may be the most cost-effective way to eliminate such a waiting list!

Aside from individual and group therapy, there are alternative formats for delivering insomnia treatment. Brief consultations and self-help treatment manuals are sometimes the only options available for individuals without insurance coverage or access to professionals with expertise in behavioral sleep medicine. A recent study by Edinger and Sampson (2003) concluded that an abbreviated 2-session intervention produced clinically meaningful benefits in about 50% of patients seen in a primary care clinic. Hauri (1993) used a brief consultation model at the Mayo Clinic and reported clinical benefits even for those patients who attended a single evaluation/therapy session. Another option is to use self-help treatment manuals, either alone or in combination with minimal professional support (Mimeault & Morin, 1999). There is no doubt that such treatment delivery is better than no treatment and is often the only option available. It may also be quite adequate for those individuals who are highly motivated and present insomnia without any other major complications. It is important to keep in mind, however, that the typical patients seen in clinical practice will need some professional support and guidance, at least during the initial phase of treatment, to implement successfully the intervention program outlined in this manual.

TREATMENT PARAMETERS: FREQUENCY, TIMING, AND DURATION OF TREATMENT

Our treatment protocol is designed to be implemented over a period of 6–10 weeks, with consultation sessions held on a weekly basis. Typically, there are one or two sessions devoted to clinical evaluation, along with a 2-week baseline sleep diary monitoring period, followed by 6–8 therapy sessions. Although both the duration of the intervention and the number of consultation sessions may vary across individuals, an average of 6 therapy sessions is necessary for most individuals with persistent insomnia. This number of sessions is needed to present a conceptual model of insomnia, describe all clinical procedures and their rationale, provide

Table 8.1. Therapy Session Agenda

- Review sleep diary.
- Evaluate compliance with clinical procedures and homework assignment.
- Identify problems during home practice and strategies for promoting treatment adherence.
- Introduce new treatment component and its rationale.
- Present didactic material supporting this component.
- Review homework assignment for the upcoming week.

enough time for patients to experiment with those procedures at home, and to problem-solve difficulties encountered during home practice. Ideally, clinical sessions are held weekly, at least during the first few weeks of therapy, to ensure continuity between sessions. If steady progress is made toward the middle of treatment, therapy visits may be held on a biweekly basis. Periodic booster sessions can also be scheduled for patients whose sleep remains fragile even after completion of the standard intervention. Obviously, treatment duration may also be extended for individuals who are more refractory to treatment and with those who present with comorbid medical conditions (e.g., chronic pain) or psychopathology (e.g., anxiety, depression). Unless it is clear that such co-existing conditions are primary and may compromise treatment outcome, we generally target the sleep problem first and, subsequently, address these concomitant dysfunctions.

The duration of therapy sessions, as well as their number, frequency and content, are likely to vary as a function of factors such as the expertise available (e.g., behavioral medicine specialist), the settings (e.g., psychology clinic vs. primary care medicine), and other practical issues (e.g., insurance coverage, etc). However, the treatment program described in this manual has been validated according to specific parameters that are outlined here. Accordingly, individual therapy sessions for insomnia typically last 50 min and group therapy sessions, which may be fewer in number, last up to 90 min. Each therapy session is highly structured and covers a different aspect of treatment. Although their specific content varies, most sessions are structured according to the agenda outlined in Table 8.1. The very first item of the agenda is to review the sleep diary for the previous week. This provides a clear message to the patient that self-monitoring is expected and is an essential component of therapy. It is useful to ask the patient to interpret his/her diary before you make your own evaluation. This exercise increases the patient's awareness of factors that may facilitate or interfere with sleep; it may also point out some interesting cognitive errors (misinterpretation, selective attention) that will become treatment targets. The next step is to check the extent to which the patient complied with your previous recommendations. Information on some of these procedures (e.g., sleep window, napping) can be directly obtained from the sleep diary but, for other procedures (e.g., getting out of bed at night), you need to rely on the patient's verbal report. The important point is to systematically review compliance with all procedures. Once adherence problems are identified, and such problems are almost always present, you need to be creative and develop concrete solutions to overcome those problems. After some problem solving, a new treatment component is introduced. Each procedure is described along with its rationale and objectives. It is important to explain how each new treatment procedure is relevant to the individual's own history of insomnia. It is also useful to provide written materials (handouts) to consolidate the new information presented during the session. The final item on the agenda is to review homework assignment for the upcoming week and, once again, a written summary should be very provided to the patient.

STRATEGIES TO PROMOTE COMPLIANCE

Throughout this manual we have endeavored to achieve ecological validity by providing vignettes or transcripts, by identifying and discussing issues pertaining to treatment implementation, and by addressing compliance more specifically at various points. This is because we recognize the importance of reflecting real clinical practice. In that real world neither patients nor therapists behave perfectly.

Indeed, the first strategy to promote compliance is to ensure that *your* practice, is best practice. The content, structure and aids to clinical appraisal and intervention in this manual have been designed with you in mind, based upon our combined experience. We would encourage you to remember that the power of any treatment lies, first and foremost, in its intrinsic effects. The evidence on CBT for insomnia is that it is an effective treatment when delivered faithfully. Treatment fidelity where the management of insomnia is concerned will invariably include the stimulus control procedures described within sleep scheduling (Chapter 5) because stimulus control has consistently been found to yield good outcomes in clinical trials. Similarly, adequate intervention must reflect the presenting needs of the patient. It seems likely, therefore, that you will need to deploy effective cognitive therapeutic methods of addressing the phenomenon of the racing mind, which is often pre-occupied with sleep or sleeplessness per se. You should bear in mind that there is limited evidence for tailoring treatment, if it is at the expense of effective therapeutic ingredients. It is attractive to match up presenting problems with treatment strategies, and

Table 8.2. Factors Likely to Be Associated with Good Compliance

---

- Provide an intervention that is evidence-based and maximize treatment fidelity.
- Establish a working relationship commensurate with the severity and intrusiveness of the problem.
- Work on problems in a focused and directed manner (using the agenda in Table 8.1).
- Monitor and discuss readiness to implement change at both the macro and micro level.
- Appraise progress collaboratively. Be prepared to persist with interventions.
- Be enthusiastic and provide encouragement.

---

this is part and parcel of experienced clinical practice, however, you should be cautious and err on the side of including components across the range of CBT strategies that we have presented. Be particularly aware that you may find it easier simply to omit components that you sense your patient may find uncomfortable or difficult to assimilate. You might be better to consider preparatory cognitive work in this situation, to overcome resistance, if your goal is to provide the most effective treatment.

In Table 8.2 we have summarized other factors that in our experience optimize compliance. You should take the patient's problem seriously by recognizing that he/she has a significant problem that is impairing their quality of life. All too often patients with insomnia are regarded as having minor complaints or symptoms of sleeplessness, rather than disorders. Bear in mind the factors we outlined in Figure 4.1. These provide the context for the consultation and the treatment sessions. The patient-therapist relationship is important in this respect. We have outlined, in Table 8.1, a suggested agenda for each session. The point here, in terms of compliance, is to be organized. CBT is a structured, rational therapy which connects between appointments as well as being internally consistent within sessions. Therapeutic work cannot be readily undertaken in, or maintained in between, sessions that lack focus or direction. Both you and your patient should be clear on what was discussed, and why, and what were agreed as action points. It is also important to identify, collaboratively, where the patient is at in terms of readiness to implement change. We encourage you to be permissive, in order to achieve an accurate appraisal of the patient's thoughts and beliefs at any point in time. If your patient is responding only to the demand characteristics of the setting, then he/she will agree to implement procedures without being ready or able to do so. If, on the other hand, the patient is acknowledging difficulty or uncertainty, you can work with that. The stages of change model (Figure 5.2) and your cognitive therapy skills are important here. Try to think of adherence and non-adherence as mental as well as behavioral states, and try to conceptualize your patient as a person with more (or less) adherence to challenge, rather than viewing compliance as a fixed trait that you either have or don't have. In many ways it is your attention to such matters that mark you out as a clinician, rather than simply a proponent of CBT for insomnia.

Table 8.2 also mentions the importance of evidence-based review. At times you will need to acknowledge that progress is limited, and some reformulation may be required. At other times, patience and perseverance may be necessary to achieve a good outcome. It is not easy to implement some of the instructions you are giving to your patients. Next time you cannot sleep try getting up after 15 minutes, perhaps 5 or 6 times in the one night It is crucial that neither you nor your patient underestimate the problem. The fact that it may take some weeks or even months to shift a disrupted sleep pattern, to let go of the 'instinct' to try to sleep, or to re-appraise the belief that day to day life is influenced by many factors other than sleep quality, is testimony to the severity and persistence of many of the insomnia problems that are out there! Finally, be enthusiastic. We are not saying that enthusiasm is therapy, but it sure helps! Patients have a right to know that the techniques you are sharing with them are effective in clinical trials, in the medium to long-term, for the majority of patients. This is good news for people who have struggled, often for many years, with a persistent insomnia. They also have a right to benefit from this knowledge. Also, although you might expect that some groups of people might do less well with CBT, there is evidence from a large scale community trial that gender, age, duration of disorder and use of hypnotic drugs were not contraindications for therapy and did not predict clinical outcome (Espie, Inglis & Harvey, 2001). In the next section, however, we will consider how you may wish to optimize your CBT intervention for particular populations.

TREATMENT OF SPECIAL POPULATIONS

There are several groups of individuals who are particularly vulnerable to suffer sleep disturbances. Among those are older adults and patients with co-existing medical conditions and psychological disorders. When insomnia is associated with another medical condition or with psychopathology, the general principle is to treat the underlying condition first. Although this initial approach is clinically sound, it is not always possible to treat effectively the associated condition, nor does this approach always resolve the concurrent sleep difficulties. For example, treatment of chronic pain or depression does not always alleviate the associated sleep disturbances. In such instances, it is necessary to directly target sleep for treatment. As we have discussed earlier, regardless of the nature of the initial triggering factors (e.g., medical, psychiatric), there are always behavioral and psychological factors contributing to perpetuate sleep disturbances over time. When managing persistent insomnia, primary or secondary in nature, the clinician should always seek to identify and modify those perpetuating factors.

The treatment protocol outlined in this manual has received extensive validation with primary insomnia. Until recently, there was little evidence of the effectiveness of such treatment for insomnia in special populations, mostly because older adults and all those patients with secondary insomnia were systematically excluded from clinical trials. Fortunately, recent studies conducted with more heterogeneous patients indicate that CBT is also effective for secondary insomnia in older adults (Lichstein, Wilson, & Johnson, 2000), as well as those whose insomnia is associated with cancer (Quesnel, Savard, Simard, Ivers, & Morin, 2003; Savard, Simard, Quesnel, Ivers, & Morin, 2002), chronic pain (Currie, Wilson, Pontefract, deLaplante, 2000), and with anxiety and depression (Morin, Stone, et al., 1994; Perlis et al., 2002). As a general rule, findings from these clinical studies indicate that baseline and endpoint scores on insomnia measures are usually more severe among patients with comorbid psychiatric and medical disorders, but the absolute changes on sleep parameters with CBT is quite comparable to results obtained by patients with primary insomnia (Morin, Stone, et al., 1994).

Of course, treatment may need to be adapted to the special needs of those populations. With older adults, for example, it is often necessary to distinguish age-related changes from pathological changes in sleep duration and quality, and adjust therapy objectives accordingly. Some behavioral procedures may also need to be adapted to circadian changes occurring with aging. Sometimes, a short nap scheduled at mid-day may be permissible to enhance alertness in the second half of the day and even to help postpone bedtime the next night. The clinician must, on the other hand, ensure that older adults maintain a regular arising time and limit the amount of time awake in bed in the morning, two factors over which retired individuals have more freedom and which may also perpetuate sleep disturbances (see Lichstein & Morin, 2000).

For patients with a medical condition such as cancer, it may be necessary to expand the scope of insomnia therapy. Whereas most of the clinical procedures remain relevant for these patients, it is essential to address other concerns (e.g., fear of death) that can directly contribute to sleep disturbances. Patients with medical conditions such as pain and cancer are often told by their treating physicians to "get plenty of rest". As such, they may spend a great deal of time lying down in bed, which may also exacerbate their sleep disturbances. You need to work around those competing recommendations and adapt some of the behavioral procedures to ensure that your patient maintain a sleep window that will provide an opportunity to get the needed rest without interfering with sleep quality. It may be necessary to incorporate additional procedures for patients to cope with daytime fatigue with other methods than bed rest (e.g., moderate exercise). Cognitive therapy is also very useful to alter some faulty beliefs and excessive concerns about the impact of lack of rest/sleep on their medical condition.

Patients with affective and anxiety disorders may also benefit from treatment targeting their sleep disturbances. Worrying and catastrophizing are cardinal features of generalized anxiety disorder and lack of sleep is often one source of this excessive worrying. With these patients, it is helpful to work on this cognitive target early on in treatment before introducing behavioral procedures. Reduced activity level and chronic rumination are also part of the clinical presentation in depression and these features need to be addressed when treating sleep disturbances. As the motivation of those patients may not be optimal for behavioral therapy, it is essential to provide additional support and encouragement to those patients. One advantage of treating insomnia early on with anxious and depressed patients is that they may generalize newly learned cognitive and behavioral skills for insomnia to other problems that may contribute to anxiety and depression.

In this chapter, we outlined several practical and clinical issues to optimize treatment implementation. We considered the advantages and limitations of individual, group, and self-help interventions, suggested some practice guidelines in terms of frequency, timing and duration of therapy, and outlined general principles to enhance treatment compliance. Although this treatment protocol is structured, sleep-focused, and evidence-based, we also firmly believe the clinician needs to remain flexible and adapt the intervention to the specific circumstances of each patient and the clinical setting in which the consultation takes place.

Appendixes

A. Outline Plan for a Sleep History Assessment Comprising Content Areas and Suggested Interview Questions

Content Area	Prompt question	Supplementary questions
Presentation of the sleep complaint		
Pattern	Can you describe the pattern of your sleep on a typical night?	Time to fall asleep? Number and duration of wakenings? Time spent asleep? Nights per week like this?
Quality	How do you feel about the quality of your sleep?	Refreshing? Enjoyable? Restless?
Daytime effects	How does your night's sleep affect your day?	Tired? Sleepy? Poor concentration? Irritable? Particular times of day?
Development of the sleep complaint	Do you remember how this spell of poor sleep started?	Events and circumstances? Dates and times? Variation since then? Exacerbating factors? Alleviating factors? Degree of impact/ intrusiveness?
Lifetime history of sleep complaints	Did you used to be a good sleeper?	Sleep in childhood? Sleep in adulthood? Nature of past episodes? Dates and times? Resolution of past episodes?

(*cont.*)

Content Area	Prompt question	Supplementary questions
General health status and medical history	Have you generally kept in good health?	Illnesses? Chronic problems? Dates and times? Recent changes in health?
Psychopathology and history of psychological functioning	Are you the kind of person who usually copes well?	Psychological problems? Anxiety or depression? Dates and times? Resourceful person? Personality type?
Issues of differential diagnosis Sleep-related breathing disorder (SBD)	Are you a heavy snorer?	Interrupted breathing in sleep? Excessively sleepy in the day?
Periodic limb movements in sleep (PLMS) and restless legs syndrome (RLS)	Do your legs sometimes twitch or can't keep still?	Excessively sleepy in the day? Trouble sitting still without moving the extremities?
Circadian rhythm sleep disorders	Do you feel you want to sleep at the wrong time?	Too early? Too late?
Parasomnias	Do you sometimes act a bit strangely during your sleep?	Behavioral description? Time during night?
Narcolepsy	Do you sometimes just fall asleep without warning?	Times and places? Collapses triggered by emotion? Poor sleep at night?
Current and previous treatments	Are you taking anything to help you sleep?	Now? In the past? Dates and times? What has worked? What have you tried yourself?

B. Sleep Diary

Instructions to patient

'This Sleep Diary is designed to provide a record of your experience of sleep, and your use of medication or alcohol to help you sleep. As you will see, information about seven nights (one week) can be recorded on one form. Please complete one column of the diary each morning, soon after you wake up. Take a few minutes to do this, trying to be as accurate as you can. It is your best estimate that we are looking for, but try not to get into the habit of clockwatching at night.'

Further instructions to clinician

At the foot of the page, there are five boxes into which you can insert the mean values for the variables sleep-onset latency (SOL: question 3), number of times of wakening from sleep (WAKE: question 4), wake time after sleep-onset (WASO: question 5), total sleep time* (TST: question 6), time in bed (TIB: question 2 minus question 1) and sleep efficiency (SE: TST divided by TIB, multiplied by 100)

---

* You may prefer to calculate TST yourself [TIB minus (SOL plus WASO)], rather than asking patients to work this out. In this case you can exclude question 6 from the Sleep Diary.

Name _____

Week Beginning _____

Measuring the Pattern of Your Sleep

	Day 1	Day 2	Day 3	Day 4	Day 5	Day 6	Day 7
1. What time did you rise from bed this morning?							
2. At what time did you go to bed last night?							
3. How long did it take you to fall asleep (minutes)?							
4. How many times did you wake up during the night?							
5. How long were you awake *during* the night (in total)?							
6. About how long did you sleep altogether (hours/mins)?							
7. How much alcohol did you take last night?							
8. How many sleeping pills did you take to help you sleep?							

Measuring the Quality of Your Sleep

1. How well do you feel this morning?
     0   1   2   3   4
   not at all moderately very							

2. How enjoyable was your sleep last night?
     0   1   2   3   4
   not at all moderately very							

For office use only

SOL	WAKE	WASO	TST	TIB	SE

C. The Insomnia Severity Index

Name:_____ Date:_____

1. Please rate the current (i.e., last 2 weeks) severity of your insomnia problem(s).

	None	Mild	Moderate	Severe	Very
a. Difficulty falling asleep:	0	1	2	3	4
b. Difficulty staying asleep:	0	1	2	3	4
c. Problem waking up too early	0	1	2	3	4

2. How satisfied/dissatisfied are you with your current sleep pattern?

Very satisfied	Satisfied	Neutral	Dissatisfied	Very dissatisfied
0	1	2	3	4

3. To what extent do you consider your sleep problem to interfere with your daily functioning (e.g. daytime fatigue, ability to function at work/daily chores, concentration, memory, mood, etc.).

Not at all interfering	A little	Somewhat	Much	Very much interfering
0	1	2	3	4

4. How noticeable to others do you think your sleeping problem is in terms of impairing the quality of your life?

Not at all noticeable	A little	Somewhat	Much	Very much noticeable
0	1	2	3	4

5. How worried/distressed are you about your current sleep problem?

Not at all worried	A little	Somewhat	Much	Very much worried
0	1	2	3	4

Guidelines for Scoring/Interpretation

Add scores for all seven items (1a + 1b + 1c + 2 + 3 + 4 + 5) =
Total score ranges from 0–28; if total score falls between:

    0–7 = No clinically significant insomnia
    8–14 = Subthreshold insomnia
    15–21 = Clinical insomnia (moderate severity)
    22–28 = Clinical insomnia (severe)

D. The Epworth Sleepiness Scale

How likely are you to doze off or fall asleep in the following situations, in contrast to feeling just tired? This refers to your usual way of life in recent times. Even if you have not done some of these things recently, try to work out how they would have affected you. Use the following scale to choose the most appropriate number for each situation.

0 = would *never* doze
1 = *slight* chance of dozing
2 = *moderate* chance of dozing
3 = *high* chance of dozing

Situation	Chance of dozing
Sitting and reading	_____
Watching TV	_____
Sitting, inactive in a public place (e.g., a theatre or a meeting)	_____
As a passenger in a car for an hour without a break	_____
Lying down in the afternoon to rest when circumstances permit	_____
Sitting and talking to someone	_____
Sitting quietly after lunch without alcohol	_____
In a car, while stopped for a few minutes in the traffic	_____

Source: M. W. Johns (1991). A new method for measuring daytime sleepiness: The Epworth Sleepiness Scale. *Sleep*, 14, 540–545. Copyright 1991 by the American Academy of Sleep Medicine. Reproduced with permission of AASM in the format Textbook via copyright Clearance Center.

E. The Pre-Sleep Arousal Scale

Instructions to patient

This scale is fairly self-explanatory. We are interested to find out about how you are feeling in your mind and in your body before you fall asleep. Please describe how intensely you experience each of the symptoms mentioned below as you attempt to fall asleep, by circling the appropriate number.

Further instructions to clinician

Two separate scores can be obtained for the PSAS. The sub-scale score for cognitive arousal comprises the total of items 1 to 8, and the sub-scale score for somatic arousal comprises the total of items 9 to 16.

	Not at all	Slightly	Moderately	A lot	Extremely
1. Worry about falling asleep	1	2	3	4	5
2. Review or ponder the events of the day	1	2	3	4	5
3. Depressing or anxious thoughts	1	2	3	4	5
4. Worry about problems other than sleep	1	2	3	4	5
5. Being mentally alert, active	1	2	3	4	5
6. Can't shut off your thoughts	1	2	3	4	5
7. Thoughts keep running through your head	1	2	3	4	5
8. Being distracted by sounds, noise in the environment	1	2	3	4	5
9. Heart racing, pounding or beating irregularly	1	2	3	4	5
10. A jittery, nervous feeling in your body	1	2	3	4	5

(continued)

	Not at all	Slightly	Moderately	A lot	Extremely
11. Shortness of breath or labored breathing	1	2	3	4	5
12. A tight, tense feeling in your muscles	1	2	3	4	5
13. Cold feeling in your hands, feet or your body in general	1	2	3	4	5
14. Have stomach upset (knot or nervous feeling in stomach, heartburn, nausea, gas, etc.)	1	2	3	4	5
15. Perspiration in palms of your hands or other parts of your body	1	2	3	4	5
16. Dry feeling in mouth or throat	1	2	3	4	5

Source: P. Nicassio, et al. The phenomenology of the pre-sleep state: The development of the Pre-Sleep Arousal Scale. *Behaviour Research and Therapy,* 23, 263–271. Copyright 1985 Elsevier. Reprinted with permission.

F. The Sleep Disturbance Questionnaire

Instructions to patient

This scale is fairly self-explanatory. We are interested to find out about the things that you feel might interfere with your sleep. Here are twelve common statements we get from people with insomnia. Take a minute or two to pick one response for each item, and then at the end write down the number of the item that you feel is most true for you

Further instructions to clinician

From our principal component analyses of the SDQ (Espie et al., 1989; 2000), we recommend summing items 1, 5, and 9 to obtain a score for "physical tension," and summing 3, 7, and 11 to obtain a score for "sleep pattern problem." The remaining items (2, 4, 6, 8, 10, 12) can be summed to obtain a score for "mental anxiety," or subdivided into "cognitive arousal" (2, 6, 10) and "sleep effort" (4, 8, 12).

On the nights when you don't sleep well the problem seems to be that (tick one box for each statement)

	Never true	Seldom true	Sometimes true	Often true	Very often true
1. I can't get into a comfortable position in bed.					
2. My mind keeps turning things over.					
3. I can't get my sleep pattern into a proper routine.					
4. I get too "worked up" at not sleeping.					
5. I find it hard to physically "let go" and relax my body.					
6. My thinking takes a long time to "unwind".					
7. I don't feel tired enough at bedtime.					

(*continued*)

	Never true	Seldom true	Sometimes true	Often true	Very often true
8. I try too hard to get to sleep.					
9. My body is full of tension					
10. I am unable to empty my mind.					
11. I spend time reading/ watching TV in bed when I should be sleeping.					
12. I worry that I won't cope tomorrow if I don't sleep well.					

Which *one* of the above statements   Number_____
   is most relevant to you?

Source: C.A. Espie et al. (1989). An evaluation of tailored psychological treatment for insomnia in terms of statistical and clinical measures of outcome. *Journal of Behaviour Therapy and Experimental Psychiatry, 20,* 143–153. Copyright Elsevier. Reprinted with permission.

G. Sleep Hygiene Practice Scale

For each cf the following behaviors, state the number of days per week (0–7) that you engage in that activity or have that experience. Base your answers on what you would consider an *average* week for yourself.

Indicate the number of days or nights in an average week you:

Days per week

1. Take a nap.
2. Go to bed hungry.
3. Go to bed thirsty.
4. Smoke more than one packet of cigarettes per day.
5. Use sleeping medications (prescribed or over the counter).
6. Drink beverages containing caffeine (e.g. coffee, tea, cola) within 4 hours of bedtime.
7. Drink more than 3 ounces of alcohol (e.g. 3 mixed drinks, 2 beers or 3 glasses of wine) within two hours of bedtime.
8. Take medications/drugs with caffeine within 4 hours of bedtime.
9. Worry as you prepare for bed about your inability to sleep.
10. Worry during the day about your inability to sleep at night.
11. Use alcohol to facilitate sleep.
12. Exercise strenuously within 2 hours of bedtime.
13. Have your sleep disturbed by light.
14. Have your sleep disturbed by noise.
15. Have your sleep disturbed by your bedpartner (put N/A if no partner).
16. Sleep approximately the same length each night.
17. Set aside time to relax before bedtime.
18. Exercise in the afternoon or early evening.
19. Have a comfortable night-time temperature in your bed/bedroom.

Source: P. Lacks, *Behavioral treatment for persistent insomnia* (1987). Copyright 1987 by Pergamon Press. Reprinted with permission.

H. Caffeine Knowledge Quiz

For each item on the following list, indicate whether you believe it contains caffeine or another stimulant by placing a Y (yes) or an N (no) in the space provided. If you are not sure, make your best guess. If you have never heard of an item please place an X in the space.

____7-Up soft drink	____lemonade	____Mountain Dew
____regular tea	____root beer	____cola soft drinks
____Dristan cold remedy	____chocolate cake	____Dexatrim diet pills
____aspirin	____regular coffee	____Tylenol
____Dr.Pepper soft drink	____Excedrin	____Aqua Ban diuretic
____Midol menstrual relief	____Sudafed decongestant	____Sprite soft drink

Source: P. Lacks (1987). *Behavioral treatment for persistent insomnia.* Copyright 1987 by Pergamon Press. Reprinted with permission.

I. Transcript of a Relaxation Therapy Session
(12-Minute Duration)

The exercises on this tape are designed to help you relax. Relaxation is a skill, which you can learn. It is just like any other skill, so don't be surprised if you find it takes practice because that is how we learn skills. So do practice. Practice a couple of times a day, especially as you start to learn. Of course, you will want to use the relaxation when you go to bed, to help you relax and go to sleep, but you will find it most useful if you have already learned what to do.

It is best to practice at a time when you know you won't be disturbed. The tape will last between ten and fifteen minutes so you will need at least that length of time set aside. When you do your relaxation exercises in your bed, you will be able to listen to the tape there too. But after a while you will have learned what to do and you will be able to just follow the exercises in your own mind.

The exercises themselves begin now.

Settle yourself down. Lie down with your hands and arms by your sides; have your eyes closed. That's good.

We will start by just thinking about your breathing. Your breathing can help you relax; the more deep and relaxed it is the better you will feel and the more in control you will feel. So begin by taking some slow regular breaths. Do that now. Breathe in fully, fill up your lungs fully; breathe in, hold your breath for a few seconds now, and let go, breathe out . . . Do that again, another deep breath, filling your lungs fully when you breathe in, hold it . . . and relax, breathe out. Continue that in your own time, noticing that each time you breathe in the muscles in your chest tighten up, and as you breathe out there is a sense of letting go. You can think the word 'relax', each time you breath out. This will remind you that breathing out helps you relax. It will also help you to use this word to tell yourself to relax whenever you need to. You will find that your body will begin to respond. Breathing slowly, comfortably, regularly, and deeply; thinking the word 'relax' every time you breath out; enjoying just lying still and having these moments to relax, concentrating on the exercises.

Now I'd like you to turn your attention to your arms and hands. At the moment just lying at your sides. I'd like you to create some tension in your hands and arms by pressing your fingers into the palms of your hands and making fists. Do that with both hands now. Feel the tension in your hands, feel the tension in your fingers and your wrists, feel the tension in your forearms. Notice what it is like. Keep it going. . .and now relax. Let those hands flop. Let them do whatever they want to do; just let them relax. Breathing slowly and deeply, you will find that your fingers will just straighten out and flop, and your hands and arms will feel more relaxed. Allow them to sink into the couch or into the bed, just allow your arms to be heavy. Breathing slowly and deeply, thinking the word 'relax' each time you breathe out, and finding that your hands and arms just relax more and more and more. Your arms and your hands so heavy and rested. It's almost as if you couldn't be bothered moving them. Just because you have let go of the energy and tension that was in the muscles there. Breathing slowly and deeply, both your hands, both your arms, heavy and rested. Let go of the energy and tension that was in the muscles there, breathing slowly and deeply. Both your hands, both your arms, heavy and rested and relaxed.

I'd like you to turn your attention now to your neck and shoulders. Again we're going to get your neck and shoulders into a state of relaxation following some tension we're going to introduce. I'd like you to do that by pulling your shoulders up towards your ears. Now, do that; pull your shoulders up towards your ears. Feel the tension across the back of your neck, across the top of your back and in your shoulders. Feel the tension, keep it going not so much that it's sore, but keep it constant. Feel it, and now let go... relax; go back to breathing slowly and deeply. Let that tension drain away, let it go. Breathe deeply, and as you do so, notice that the tension, almost like a stream, drains away from your neck, across your shoulders, down the upper part of your arms, down the lower part of your arms and out through your fingertips. Draining out and leaving a sense of warmth and relaxation deep in your muscles. Breathing slowly and deeply and allowing that to take place. Just let the tension go. If it doesn't seem to go, don't force it, it will go itself. Be confident about that. Just breathe slowly and deeply and allow yourself to be relaxed; remembering to think the word 'relax', each time you breathe out. Using that word 'relax' to focus on the sense of relaxation that you get, using the word 'relax' to remind you of the success your are having in relaxing your body.

I'd like you to concentrate now on your face, and on your jaw, and on your forehead. I'd like you to create some tension in these parts of your body by doing two things together at the same time. These things are to screw up your eyes really tightly and bite your teeth together. Do these things together now. Bite your teeth together; feel the tension in your jaw. Screw up your eyes; feel the tension all around your eyes, in your forehead, in your cheeks, throughout your face, wherever there is tension. Now keep it going... and relax; breathing in through your nose and out through your mouth, slowly and deeply. Notice how your forehead smoothes out and then your eyelids and your cheeks. Allow your jaw to hang slightly open. Allow your whole head to feel heavy and to sink into the pillow; breathing slowly and deeply. Allow there to be a spread of relaxation across the surface of your face and into all those muscles in your face. Allow your eyelids to feel heavy and comfortable, your jaw and your whole head; breathing slowly and deeply, enjoying the relaxation which you feel in your body. Relax each time you breathe out. Relax just that little bit more each time you breathe out".

Concentrating now on your legs and feet, I want you to create some tension here by doing two things at the same time; and these things are to press the backs of your legs downwards and to pull your toes back towards your head. Do these things together now. Create the tension in your legs, press the backs of your legs downwards and pull your toes back towards your head. Feel the tension in your feet, in your toes, in your ankles, in the muscles in your legs. Feel what it is like. Don't overdo it; just notice what it is like . . . and relax. Breathing slowly and deeply once more; just allow your feet to flop any old way. Allow the muscles to give up their energy, give up their tension. Let it go, breathing slowly and deeply. Notice how your feet just want to flop to the side. Notice how your legs feel heavy as if you couldn't be bothered moving them. Heavy and comfortable and rested and relaxed. Just that little bit more relaxed each time you breathe out.

Be thinking about your whole body now; supported by the bed, sinking into it, but supported by it. You've let go the tension throughout your body. Your body feels rested, comfortable. Enjoy each deep breath you take. Just use these few moments now to think about any part of your body that doesn't feel quite so rested and allow the tension to go. It will go. Breathe slowly and deeply; thinking the word 'relax' each time you breathe out. Just let any remaining tension drain away; from your hands, your arms, your neck and your back. Heavy and rested, comfortable and relaxed. From your face and your eyes, from your forehead; letting the muscles give up their energy. Like a stream of relaxation flowing over your whole body. Let your legs and feet feel relaxed; sinking into the bed. Breathing slowly and deeply.

In a few moments, this tape will finish; but you can continue to relax. You may wish to repeat some of the exercises yourself and that is fine. You may wish to enjoy just continuing as your are. You may wish to think on your visualization scene or build pictures in your mind that will help you to relax further. It's up to you, but continue to relax.

The tape itself stops now.

J. The Sleep Behavior Self-Rating Scale

Instructions for patients

This rating scale helps us to understand what your behavior pattern around bedtime is like. It is fairly self-explanatory. Please take a few minutes to fill it in as accurately as you can. Please indicate how often you do the following things *in your bed before falling asleep* or *while in your bedroom*. Complete the form by considering what you would do in an average week.

Behavior	Never	Rarely	Sometimes	Often	Very often
Read a book or magazine					
Watch TV					
Listen to the radio					
Have a conversation with someone					
Speak on the telephone					
Eat or drink					
Smoke					
Please also answer the following questions:					
I take naps during the day or evening					
I feel sleepy when I go to bed					
I switch the light off as soon as I get into bed					
I spend a lot of time lying awake in bed at night					
If I can t get to sleep within approx. 20 minutes I get out of bed and move to another room until I feel sleepy again					
I set myself a regular rising time each morning					
If I have a bad night's sleep I still get up at my usual time					

Source: Adapted from S.S. Kazarian, M.G. Howe, and K.G. Csapo (1979). Development of the Sleep Behavior Self-Rating Scale. *Behavior Therapy, 10*, 412–417. Copyright 1979 by the Association for Advancement of Behavior Therapy. Reprinted by permission of the publisher.

K. Summary of the Sleep Scheduling Treatment Program

Instructions to clinician

You can reproduce this summary sheet as a handout to give to your patients. Bear in mind the implementation issues described in the text and in Table 5.3.

1. Work out your current average sleep time and plan to spend that amount of time in bed.
2. Decide on a set rising time to get up each morning and put that into practice.
3. Establish a threshold time for going to be by subtracting sleep time from rising time, and stay out of bed until your threshold time.
4. Lie down intending to go to sleep only when you feel sleepy at or after the threshold time.
5. Follow this program seven days/nights a week.
6. If you do not sleep within 15 minutes get up and go into another room. Do something relaxing and go back to bed when you feel sleepy again. Repeat this if you still cannot sleep or if you waken during the night.
7. Adjust the new schedule by a maximum of 15 minutes per week, dependent upon your sleep efficiency.
8. Do not use your bed for anything except sleep (and sexual activity) and turn the light out when you go to bed.
9. Do not nap during the day or evening.

L. Calculating Current Sleep Requirement for Sleep Restriction

First, write down in the spaces below the amount of time you think you actually slept on each of the last 10 nights, from your Sleep Diary (it may be easier to convert the time to the total number of minutes per night.)

Second, add up the total time you have slept across these nights.

Third, divide the total by 10 to get the average length of your night's sleep.

Night   Amount Slept

   1.

   2.

   3.

   4.

   5.

   6.

   7.

   8.

   9.

  10.

Total amount of time over 10 days = _____

Average sleep time = _____/10 = _____

M. Self-Monitoring Form of Sleep-Related Thoughts

Situation	Automatic thoughts	Emotions
Watching TV in the evening	"I must get some sleep tonight, I have so much to do tomorrow"	Anxious 80%

N. Dysfunctional Beliefs and Attitudes about Sleep Scale

Instructions to patient

Several statements reflecting people's beliefs and attitudes about sleep are listed below. Please indicate to what extent you personally agree or disagree with each statement. There is no right or wrong answer. For each statement circle the number that corresponds to your own *personal belief*. Please respond to all items even though some may not apply directly to your own situation.

Strongly disagree										Strongly agree
0	1	2	3	4	5	6	⑦	8	9	10

1. I need 8 hours of sleep to feel refreshed and function well during the day.

0	1	2	3	4	5	6	7	8	9	10

2. When I don't get proper amount of sleep on a given night, I need to catch up on the next day by napping or on the next night by sleeping longer.

0	1	2	3	4	5	6	7	8	9	10

3. Because I am getting older, I need less sleep.

0	1	2	3	4	5	6	7	8	9	10

4. I am worried that if I go for 1 or 2 nights without sleep, I may have a "nervous breakdown."

0	1	2	3	4	5	6	7	8	9	10

5. I am concerned that chronic insomnia may have serious consequences on my physical health.

0	1	2	3	4	5	6	7	8	9	10

6. By spending more time in bed, I usually get more sleep and feel better the next day.

| 0 | 1 | 2 | 3 | 4 | 5 | 6 | 7 | 8 | 9 | 10 |

7. When I have trouble falling asleep or getting back to sleep after nighttime awakening, I should stay in bed and try harder.

| 0 | 1 | 2 | 3 | 4 | 5 | 6 | 7 | 8 | 9 | 10 |

8. I am worried that I may lose control over my abilities to sleep.

| 0 | 1 | 2 | 3 | 4 | 5 | 6 | 7 | 8 | 9 | 10 |

9. Because I am getting older, I should go to bed earlier in the evening.

| 0 | 1 | 2 | 3 | 4 | 5 | 6 | 7 | 8 | 9 | 10 |

10. After a poor night's sleep, I know that it will interfere with my daily activities on the next day.

| 0 | 1 | 2 | 3 | 4 | 5 | 6 | 7 | 8 | 9 | 10 |

11. In order to be alert and function well during the day, I believe I would be better off taking a sleeping pill rather than having a poor night's sleep.

| 0 | 1 | 2 | 3 | 4 | 5 | 6 | 7 | 8 | 9 | 10 |

12. When I feel irritable, depressed, or anxious during the day, it is mostly because I did not sleep well the night before.

| 0 | 1 | 2 | 3 | 4 | 5 | 6 | 7 | 8 | 9 | 10 |

13. Because my bed partner falls asleep as soon as his/her head hits the pillow and stays asleep through the night, I should be able to do so too.

| 0 | 1 | 2 | 3 | 4 | 5 | 6 | 7 | 8 | 9 | 10 |

14. I feel that insomnia is basically the result of aging and there isn't much that can be done about this problem.

| 0 | 1 | 2 | 3 | 4 | 5 | 6 | 7 | 8 | 9 | 10 |

15. I am sometimes afraid of dying in my sleep.

| 0 | 1 | 2 | 3 | 4 | 5 | 6 | 7 | 8 | 9 | 10 |

16. When I have a good night's sleep, I know that I will have to pay for it on the following night.

| 0 | 1 | 2 | 3 | 4 | 5 | 6 | 7 | 8 | 9 | 10 |

17. When I sleep poorly on one night, I know it will disturb my sleep schedule for the whole week.

| 0 | 1 | 2 | 3 | 4 | 5 | 6 | 7 | 8 | 9 | 10 |

18. Without an adequate night's sleep, I can hardly function the next day.

| 0 | 1 | 2 | 3 | 4 | 5 | 6 | 7 | 8 | 9 | 10 |

19. I can't ever predict whether I'll have a good or poor night's sleep.

| 0 | 1 | 2 | 3 | 4 | 5 | 6 | 7 | 8 | 9 | 10 |

20. I have little ability to manage the negative consequences of disturbed sleep.

| 0 | 1 | 2 | 3 | 4 | 5 | 6 | 7 | 8 | 9 | 10 |

21. When I feel tired, have no energy, or just seem not to function well during the day, it is generally because I did not sleep well the night before.

| 0 | 1 | 2 | 3 | 4 | 5 | 6 | 7 | 8 | 9 | 10 |

22. I get overwhelmed by my thoughts at night and often feel I have no control over this racing mind.

| 0 | 1 | 2 | 3 | 4 | 5 | 6 | 7 | 8 | 9 | 10 |

23. I feel I can still lead a satisfactory life despite sleep difficulties.

| 0 | 1 | 2 | 3 | 4 | 5 | 6 | 7 | 8 | 9 | 10 |

24. I believe insomnia is essentially the result of a chemical imbalance.

| 0 | 1 | 2 | 3 | 4 | 5 | 6 | 7 | 8 | 9 | 10 |

25. I feel insomnia is ruining my ability to enjoy life and prevents me from doing what I want.

| 0 | 1 | 2 | 3 | 4 | 5 | 6 | 7 | 8 | 9 | 10 |

26. A "nightcap" before bedtime is a good solution to sleep problem.

| 0 | 1 | 2 | 3 | 4 | 5 | 6 | 7 | 8 | 9 | 10 |

27. Medication is probably the only solution to sleeplessness.

| 0 | 1 | 2 | 3 | 4 | 5 | 6 | 7 | 8 | 9 | 10 |

28. My sleep is getting worse all the time and I don't believe anyone can help.

| 0 | 1 | 2 | 3 | 4 | 5 | 6 | 7 | 8 | 9 | 10 |

29. It usually shows in my physical appearance when I haven't slept well.

| 0 | 1 | 2 | 3 | 4 | 5 | 6 | 7 | 8 | 9 | 10 |

30. I avoid or cancel obligations (social, family) after a poor night's sleep.

| 0 | 1 | 2 | 3 | 4 | 5 | 6 | 7 | 8 | 9 | 10 |

Scoring and interpretation guidelines

The total DBAS score is obtained by adding the score of each item (reverse score for item 23) and dividing by the total number of items. The are no norms available for this scale but a higher score indicates that your patient endorses more intense and more frequent dysfunctional beliefs and attitudes about sleep.

An abbreviated 16-item version is currently under validation.

O. Example of an Automatic Thought Record Used for Cognitive Therapy

Situation	Automatic thoughts	Emotions	Alternative thoughts	Emotions
Awake in bed in the middle of the night	"I won't be able to function tomorrow"	Anxious 80%	"There is no point in worrying about this now. Sometimes I can still function after a poor night's sleep".	Anxious 25%

P. The Glasgow Content of Thoughts Inventory

Instructions to patient

This is a brief measure which should only take you a few minutes to complete. We are interested in the types of thoughts that you have while you are trying to get to sleep. Many people with insomnia complain of a 'racing mind' or of thoughts that seem to get in the way of falling asleep. Simply mark one of the boxes for each of the items on the scale as an indication of how often this particular thought has been a problem for you during the past week.

Further instructions to clinician

The GITI is scored by adding up responses to give a total score for thought intrusion 'Never' is scored 1, 'sometimes' 2, 'often' 3 and 'always' 4. Our preliminary work suggests that a score of 42 yields a sensitivity of 100% and a specificity of 83% in discriminating between insomniacs and good sleepers (Harvey & Espie, 2003). Principal component analysis identified 3 subscales – 'cognitive intrusions relating to active problem-solving (items 1, 3, 8, 12, 14, 15, 19, 21 and 23), 'cognitive intrusions relating to sleep and wakefulness' (items 5, 6, 7, 9, 11, 18, 22, 24, and 25) and 'cognitive intrusions relating to somatic and sensory engagement' (items 2, 4, 10, 13, 16, 17, and 20). You may find it helpful also to calculate this subscale profile to identify in which area(s) the main intrusions fall.

	Never	Sometimes	Often	Always
1. Things in the future				
2. How tired/sleepy you feel				
3. Things that happened that day				
4. How nervous/anxious you feel				
5. How mentally awake you feel				
6. Checking the time				
7. Trivial things				
8. How you can't stop your mind from racing				
9. How long you've been awake				
10. Your health				
11. Ways you can get to sleep				
12. Things you have to do tomorrow				
13. How hot/cold you feel				

(continued)

169

	Never	Sometimes	Often	Always
14. Your work/responsibilities				
15. How frustrated/annoyed you feel				
16. How light/dark the room is				
17. Noises you hear				
18. Being awake all night				
19. Pictures in your mind				
20. The effects of not sleeping well				
21. Your personal life				
22. How thinking too much is the problem				
23. Things in your past				
24. How bad you are at sleeping				
25. Things to do to help you sleep				

Q. The Glasgow Sleep Effort Scale

The following seven statements relate to your night-time sleep pattern *in the past week*. Please indicate by circling *one* response how true each statement is for you

1. I put too much effort into sleeping at night when it should come naturally

   Very much   To some extent   Not at all

2. I feel I should be able to control my sleep at night

   Very much   To some extent   Not at all

3. I put off going to bed at night for fear of not being able to sleep

   Very much   To some extent   Not at all

4. I worry about not sleeping if I am in bed at night and cannot sleep

   Very much   To some extent   Not at all

5. I am no good at sleeping at night

   Very much   To some extent   Not at all

6. I get anxious about sleeping before I go to bed at night

   Very much   To some extent   Not at all

7. I worry about the long term consequences of not sleeping at night

   Very much   To some extent   Not at all

R. A Medication Withdrawal Schedule Form

Week	Type	Dosage (mg)	Number of nights	Total amount (mg)	% dosage reduction	Self-efficacy (0–100%)
Baseline						
Week 1						
Week 2						
Week 3						
Week 4						
Week 5						
Week 6						
Week 7						
Week 8						
Week 9						
Week 10						

References

American Psychiatric Association (1990). *Benzodiazepine dependence, toxicity, and abuse: A task force report of the American Psychiatric Association.* Washington DC: American Psychiatric Association.

American Psychiatric Association (1994). *Diagnostic and Statistical Manual of Mental Disorders* (DSM-IV). Washington DC: American Psychiatric Association.

American Sleep Disorders Association (1995a). Practice parameters for the use of polysomnography in the evaluation of insomnia. *Sleep, 18,* 55–57.

American Sleep Disorders Association (1995b). Practice parameters for the use of actigraphy in the clinical assessment of sleep disorders. *Sleep, 18,* 285–287.

American Sleep Disorders Association (1997). *International Classification of Sleep Disorders: Diagnostic and Coding Manual.* Revised ed. Rochester, MN: American Sleep Disorders Association.

Ansfield, M.E., Wegner, D.M., & Bowser, R. (1996). Ironic effects of sleep urgency. *Behaviour Research and Therapy, 34,* 523–531.

Ashton, H. (1994). The treatment of benzodiazepine dependence. *Addiction, 89,* 1535–1541.

Ascher, L.M. & Turner, R.M. (1979). Paradoxical intention and insomnia: An experimental investigation. *Behaviour Research and Therapy, 17,* 408–11.

Baillargeon, L., Landreville, P., Verreault, R., Beauchemin, J-P., Grégoire, J-P., & Morin, C.M. (in press). Discontinuation of benzodiazepines among older insomniac adults treated through cognitive-behavioral therapy combined with gradual tapering: A randomized trial. *Canadian Medical Association Journal.*

Bastien, C. Vallières, A. & Morin, C. M. (2001). Validation of the Insomnia Severity Index as a clinical outcome measure for insomnia research. *Sleep Medicine, 2,* 297–307.

Bastien, C. Vallières, A. & Morin, C. M. (In press). Precipitating factors of insomnia. *Behavioral Sleep Medicine.*

Beck, J.A. (1995). *Cognitive therapy: Basics and beyond.* New York: Guilford Press.

Billard, M. (1994). *Le sommeil normal et pathologique. [Normal and pathological sleep].* Paris: Masson.

Billiard, M., Besset, A. & Cadilhac, J. (1983). The clinical and polygraphic development of narcolepsy (pp. 187–199). In C. Guilleminault & E. Lugaresi (Eds). *Sleep/wake disorders: natural history, epidemiology and long-term evaluation.* New York: Raven Press.

Blood, M.L., Sack, R.L., Percy, D.S., & Pen, J.C. (1997). A comparison of sleep detection by wrist actigraphy, behavioral response, and polysomnography. *Sleep, 20,* 388–395.

Bonnet, M.H. (2000). Sleep deprivation. In M. Kryger, T. Roth, W. Dement (Eds.), *Principles and practice of sleep medicine* (3rd. Ed., pp. 53–71). Philadelphia, Pa: W.B. Saunders.

Bonnet, M.H. & Arand, D.L. (1992). Caffeine use as a model of acute and chronic insomnia. *Sleep, 15,* 526–536.

Bonnet, M.H. & Arand, D.L. (1995). 24 hour metabolic rate in insomniacs and matched normal sleepers. *Sleep, 18,* 581–588.

Bootzin, R.R. (1972). A stimulus control treatment for insomnia. *Proceedings of the American Psychological Association,* 395–396.

Bootzin, R.R. & Epstein, D.R. (2000). Stimulus control (pp. 167–184). In K.L. Lichstein, & C.M. Morin (Eds). *Treatment of late-life insomnia.* Thousand Oaks, Ca.: Sage Publications.

Bootzin, R.R., Epstein, D., & Wood, J.M. (1991). Stimulus control instructions (pp. 19–28). In P.J. Hauri (Ed.). *Case studies in insomnia.* New York: Plenum Press.

Bootzin, R.R. & Rider, S.P. (1997). Behavioural techniques and biofeedback for insomnia (pp. 315–328). In Pressman, M.R. & W.C. Orr (Eds). *Understanding sleep. The evaluation and treatment of sleep disorders.* Washington DC: American Psychological Association.

Borbely, A.A. (1994). Sleep homeostasis and models of sleep regulation (pp. 309–320). In M.H., Kryger, T., Roth & W.C., Dement (Eds.). *Principles and practice of sleep medicine* (2nd edition). Philadelphia, Pa.: WB Saunders Company.

Breslau, N., Roth, T., Rosenthal, L., & Andreski, P. (1996). Sleep disturbance and psychiatric disorders: A longitudinal epidemiological study of young adults. *Biological Psychiatry, 39,* 411–418.

Broman, J.E. & Hetta, J. (1994). Perceived pre-sleep arousal in patients with persistent psychophysiologic and psychiatric insomnia. *Nordic Journal of Psychiatry, 48,* 203–207.

Busto, U.E., Sellers, E.M., Naranjo, C.A., Cappell, H., Sanchez-Craig, M., & Sykora, K. (1986). Withdrawal reactions after long-term therapeutic use of benzodiazepines. *New England Journal of Medecine, 315,* 854–859.

Buysse, D.J. & Reynolds, C.R. (2000). Pharmacologic treatment. In K.L. Lichstein and C.M. Morin (Eds.), *Treatment of late-life insomnia* (pp. 231–267). Thousand Oaks, CA: Sage Publications.

Buysse, D.J., Reynolds, C.F., Kupfer, D.J., Thorpy, M.J., Bixler, E., Manfredi, R., et al. (1994). Clinical diagnoses in 216 insomnia patients using the international classification of sleep disorders (ICSD), DSM-IV and ICD-10 categories: A report from the APA/NIMH DSM-IV field trial. *Sleep, 17,* 630–637.

Buysse, D.J., Reynolds, C.F., Monk, T.H., Berman, S.R., & Kupfer, D.J. (1989). The Pittsburgh Sleep Quality Index: A new instrument for psychiatric practice and research. *Psychiatry Research, 28,* 193–213.

Buysse, D.J., Reynolds, C.F., Kupfer, D.J., Thorpy, M.J., Bixler, E., Kales, A., et al. (1997). Effects of diagnosis on treatment recommendations in chronic insomnia—A report from the APA/NIMH DSM-IV field trial. *Sleep, 20*, 542–552.

Carskadon, M.A. & Dement, W.C. (2000). Normal human sleep: An overview. In M. Kryger, T. Roth, & W. Dement (Eds.), *Principles and practice of sleep medicine* (3rd. Ed., pp. 15–25). Philadelphia, Pa: W.B. Saunders.

Carskadon, M.A. & Dement, W.C. (1981). Cumulative effects of sleep restriction on daytime sleepiness. *Psychophysiology, 18*, 107–113.

Carskadon, M.A., Dement, W.C., Mitler, M.M., Roth, T., & Westbrook, P.R. (1986). Guidelines for the multiple sleep latency test (MSLT): A standard measure of sleepiness. *Sleep, 9*, 519–524.

Chesson, A.L., Ferber, R.A., Fry, J.M., Grigg-Damberger, M., Hartse, K.M., Hurwitz, T.D., et al. (1997). The indications for polysomnography and related procedures. *Sleep, 20*, 423–487.

Chesson, A.L., Hartse, K., Anderson, W.M., Davila, D., Johnson, S., Littner, M., et al. (2000). Practice parameters for the evaluation of chronic insomnia. *Sleep, 23*, 237–241.

Chesson, A.L., Anderson, W.M., Littner, M., Davila, D., Hartse, K., Hurwitz, T.D., et al. (1999). Practice parameters for the nonpharmacologic treatment of chronic insomnia. *Sleep, 22*, 1128–1133.

Culebras, A. & Magana, R. (1987). Neurologic disorders and sleep disturbances. *Seminars in Neurology, 7*, 277–285.

Currie, S.R., Wilson, K.G., Pontefract, A.J., & deLaplante, L. (2000). Cognitive-behavioral treatment of insomnia secondary to chronic pain. *Journal of Consulting and Clinical Psychology, 68*, 407–416.

Czeisler, C.A. & Khalsa, S.B.S. (2000). The human circadian timing system and sleep-wake regulation. In M. Kryger, T. Roth, W. Dement (Eds.), *Principles and practice of sleep medicine* (3rd. Ed., pp. 353–375). Philadelphia, PA: W.B. Saunders.

Dinges, D.F. (1995). An overview of sleepiness and accidents. *Journal of Sleep Research, 4*, 4–14.

DuPont, R.L. (1990). A practical approach to benzodiazepine discontinuation. *Journal of Psychiatric Research, 24*, 81–90.

Edinger, J.D. & Fins, A.I. (1995). The distribution and clinical significance of sleep time misperceptions among insomniacs. *Sleep, 18*, 232–239.

Edinger, J.D., Fins, A.I., Sullivan, R.J., Marsh, G.R., Dailey, D.S., Hope, T.V., et al. (1997). Sleep in the laboratory and sleep at home: comparisons of older insomniacs and normal sleepers. *Sleep, 20*, 1119–1126.

Edinger, J.D. & Sampson, W.S. (2003). A primary care "friendly" cognitive behavioral insomnia therapy. *Sleep, 26*, 177–182.

Edinger, J.D., Sullivan, R.J., Bastian, L.A., Hope, T.V., Young, M., Shaw, E., et al. (2000). Insomnia and the eye of the beholder: Are there clinical markers of objective sleep disturbances among adults with and without insomnia complaints? *Journal of Consulting and Clinical Psychology, 68*, 586–593.

Edinger, J.D., Wohlgemuth, W.K., Radtke, R.A., Marsh, G.R., & Quillian, R.E. (2001a). Does cognitive-behavioral insomnia therapy alter dysfunctional beliefs about sleep? *Sleep, 24*, 591–599.

Edinger, J.D., Wohlgemuth, W. K., Radtke, R. A. Marsh, G.R., Quillian, R.E. (2001b). Cognitivie behavioral therapy for treatment of chronic primary insomnia: A randomized controlled trial. *Journal of the American Medical Association, 285*, 1856–1864.

Espie, C.A. (1991). *The psychological treatment of insomnia.* Chichester, United Kingdom: Wiley.

Espie, C.A. (2002). Insomnia: Conceptual issues in the development, persistence, and treatment of sleep disorders in adults. *Annual Review of Psychology, 53*, 215–243.

Espie, C.A., Brooks, D.N. & Lindsay, W.R. (1989). An evaluation of tailored psychological treatment for insomnia in terms of statistical and clinical measures of outcome. *Journal of Behaviour Therapy and Experimental Psychiatry, 20*, 143–153.

Espie, C.A., Inglis, S.J., Harvey, L., & Tessier, S. (2000). Insomniacs' attributions: Psychometric properties of the Dysfunctional Beliefs and Attitudes about Sleep scale and the Sleep Disturbance Questionnaire. *Journal of Psychosomatic Research, 48*, 141–148.

Espie, C.A., Inglis, S.J., & Harvey, L. (2001). Predicting clinically significant response to cognitive behavior therapy (CBT) for chronic insomnia in general practice: Analyses of outcome data at 12 months post-treatment. *Journal of Consulting and Clinical Psychology, 69*, 58–66.

Espie, C.A., Inglis, S.J., Tessier, S., & Harvey, L. (2001). The clinical effectiveness of cognitive behaviour therapy for chronic insomnia: Implementation and evaluation of a *sleep clinic* in general medical practice. *Behaviour Research and Therapy, 39*, 45–60.

Espie, C.A. & Lindsay, W.R. (1985). Paradoxical intention in the treatment of chronic insomnia: Six cases illustrating variability in therapeutic response. *Behaviour Research and Therapy, 23*, 703–709.

Espie, C.A. & Lindsay, W.R. (1987). Cognitive strategies for the management of severe sleep-maintenance insomnia: A preliminary investigation. *Behavioural Psychotherapy, 15*, 388–395.

Espie, C.A., Lindsay, W.R., & Brooks, N. (1988). Substituting behavioural treatment for drugs in the treatment of insomnia: An exploratory study. *Journal of Behavior Therapy and Experimental Psychiatry, 19*, 51–56.

Espie, C.A, Lindsay, W.R., Brooks, D.N., Hood, E.H., & Turvey, T. (1989). A controlled comparative investigation of psychological treatments for chronic insomnia. *Behaviour Research and Therapy, 27*, 51–56.

Espie, C.A., Lindsay, W.R., & Espie, L.C. (1989). Use of the Sleep Assessment Device (Kelley & Lichstein, 1980) to validate insomniacs' self-report of sleep pattern. *Journal of Psychopathology and Behavioral Assessment, 11*, 71–79.

Fichten, C.S., Libman, E., Creti, L., Amsel, R., Tagalakis, V., & Brender, W. (1998). Thoughts during awake times in older good and poor sleepers: The Self-Statement Test 60+. *Cognitive Therapy and Research, 22*, 1–20.

Ford, D.E. & Kamerow, D.B. (1989). Epidemiologic study of sleep disturbances and psychiatric disorders: An opportunity for prevention? *Journal of the American Medical Association, 262*, 1479–1484.

Fraser, D., Peterkin, G.S., Gamsu, C.V., & Baldwin, P.J. (1990). Benzodiazepine withdrawal: A pilot comparison of three methods. *British Journal of Clinical Psychology, 29*, 231–233.

Freedman, R.R. & Sattler, H.L. (1982). Physiological and psychological factors in sleep-onset insomnia. *Journal of Abnormal Psychology, 91*, 380–389.

Freeman, A., Pretzer, J., Fleming, B., & Simon, K.M. (1990). *Clinical applications of cognitive therapy.* New York: Plenum Press.

Gillin, J.C._ Spinweber, C.L., & Johnson, L.C. (1989). Rebound insomnia: A critical review. *Journal of Clinical Psychopharmacology, 9*, 161–172.

Greenblatt. D.J. (1991). Benzodiazepine hypnotics: Sorting the pharmacokinetic facts. *The Journal of Clinical Psychiatry, 52* (Suppl.), 4–10.

Haimov, I. & Lavie, P. (1997). Circadian characteristics of sleep propensity function in healthy elderly: A comparison with young adults. *Sleep, 20*, 294–300.

Hajak, G. 2002). Zolpidem "as needed" versus continuous administration: Pan-European study results. *Sleep Medicine Reviews, 6* (Suppl. 1), S21–S28.

Harvey, A.G. (2000a). Sleep hygiene and sleep-onset insomnia. *Journal of Nervous and Mental Disease, 188*, 53–55.

Harvey, A.G. (2000b). Pre-sleep cognitive activity in insomnia: A comparison of sleep-onset insomniacs and good sleepers. *British Journal of Clinical Psychology, 39*, 275–286.

Harvey, A.G. (in press). Attempted suppression of pre-sleep cognitive activity in insomnia. *Cognitive Research and Therapy.*

Harvey A.G., & Payne, S. (2002). The management of unwanted pre-sleep thoughts in insomnia: distraction with imagery versus general distraction. *Behaviour Research & Therapy, 40*, 267–277.

Harvey, L., & Espie, C.A. (2001). Putative models of insomnia: A comparative study of primary insomniacs, depressed insomniacs and good sleepers. Unpublished doctoral thesis, University of Glasgow.

Harvey, K.J., & Espie, C.A. (in press). Development and preliminary validation of the Glasgow Content of Thoughts Inventory (GCTI): A new measure of the assessment of pre-sleep cognitive activity. *British Journal of Clinical Psychology.*

Hauri, P.J. (1993). Consulting about insomnia: A method and some preliminary data. *Sleep, 16*, 340–350.

Hauri, P.J. (1997). Insomnia: Can we mix behavioral therapy with hypnotics when treating insomniacs? *Sleep, 20*, 1111–1118.

Hauri, P.J. & Fisher, J. (1986). Persistent psychophysiologic (learned) insomnia. *Sleep, 9*, 38–53.

Hauri, P.J. & Wisbey, J. (1992). Wrist actigraphy in insomnia. *Sleep, 15*, 293–301.

Hoch, C.C., Dew, M.A., Reynolds, C.F., Buysse, D.J., Noel, P.D., Monk, T.H., et al. (1997). Longitudinal changes in diary- and laboratory-based sleep measures in healthy "old old" and "young old" subjects: A three year follow up. *Sleep, 20*, 192–202.

Hohagen, F., Montero, R.F., Weiss, E., Lis, S., Schonbrunn, E., Dressing, H., et al. (1994). Treatment of primary insomnia with trimipramine: An alternative to benzodiazepine hypnotics? *European Archives of Psychiatry and Clinical Neuroscience, 244*, 65–72.

Holbrook, A.M., Crowther, R., Lotter, A., Cheng, C., & King, D. (2000). Meta-analysis of benzodiazepine use in the treatment of insomnia. *Canadian Medical Association Journal, 162,* 225–233.

Horne, J.A. (1988). Why we sleep: The functions of sleep in humans and other mammals. Oxford: Oxford University Press.

Johns, M.W. (1991). A new method for measuring daytime sleepiness: The Epworth Sleepiness Scale. *Sleep, 14,* 540–545.

Katz, D.A. & McHorney, C.A. (1988). Clinical correlates of insomnia in patients with chronic illness. *Archives of Internal Medicine, 158,* 1099–1107.

Kazarian, S.S., Howe, M.G. & Csapo, K.G. (1979). Development of the Sleep Behaviour Self-Rating Scale. *Behavior Therapy, 10,* 412–417.

Kirmil-Gray, K., Eagleston, J.R., Thorensen, C.E., & Zarcone, V.P. (1985). Brief consultation and stress management treatments for drug-dependent insomnia: Effects on sleep quality, self-efficacy, and daytime stress. *Journal of Behavioral Medicine, 8,* 79–99.

Lacks, P. (1987). *Behavioral treatment for persistent insomnia.* New York: Pergamon Press.

Lacks, P. & Rotert, M. (1986). Knowledge and practice of sleep hygiene techniques in insomniacs and good sleepers. *Behaviour Research and Therapy, 24,* 365–368.

Lader, M.H. (1990). Benzodiazepine withdrawal. In R. Noyes, M. Roth & G.D. Burrows (Eds.), *Handbook of anxiety* (pp. 57–71). Amsterdam, Netherlands: Elsevier.

Levey, A.B., Aldaz, J.A., Watts, F.N., & Coyle, K. (1991). Articulatory suppression and the treatment of insomnia. *Behaviour Research and Therapy, 29,* 85–89.

Lichstein, K.L. & Johnson, R.S. (1991). Older adults' objective self-recording of sleep in the home. *Behavior Therapy, 22,* 531–549.

Lichstein, K.L. & Johnson, R.S. (1993). Relaxation for insomnia and hypnotic medication use in older women. *Psychology and Aging, 8,* 103–111.

Lichstein, K.L. & Morin, C.M. (2000). *Treatment of late life insomnia.* Thousand Oaks, Ca.: Sage Publications.

Lichstein, K.L., Peterson, B.A., Riedel, B.W., Means, M.K., Epperson, M.T., & Aguillard, R.N. (1999). Relaxation to assist sleep medication withdrawal. *Behavior Modification, 23,* 379–402.

Lichstein, K.L. & Riedel, B.W. (1994). Behavioral assessment and treatment of insomnia: A review with an emphasis on clinical application. *Behavior Therapy, 25,* 659–688.

Lichstein, K.L., Riedel, B.W., Lester, K.W., & Aguillard, R.N. (1999). Occult sleep apnea in a recruited sample of older adults with insomnia. *Journal of Consulting and Clinical Psychology, 67,* 405–410.

Lichstein, K.L. & Rosenthal, T.L. (1980). Insomniacs' perceptions of cognitive versus somatic determinants of sleep disturbance. *Journal of Abnormal Psychology, 89,* 105–107.

Lichstein, K.L., Wilson, N.M., & Johnson, C.T. (2000). Psychological treatment of secondary insomnia. *Psychology and Aging, 15,* 232–240.

McClusky, H.Y., Milby, J.B., Switzer, P.K., Williams, V., & Wooten, V. (1991). Efficacy of behavioral versus triazolam treatment in persistent sleep-onset insomnia. *American Journal of Psychiatry, 148,* 121–126.

Mendelsor, W.B. (1997). A critical evaluation of the hypnotic efficacy of melatonin. *Sleep, 20*, 916–919.

Merica, H. Blois R., & Gaillard, J.M. (1998). Spectral characteristics of sleep EEG in chronic insomnia. *European Journal of Neurosciences, 10*, 1826–1834.

Milby, J.B. Williams, V., Hall, J.N., Khuder, S., McGill, T., & Wooten, V. (1993). Effectiveness of combined triazolam-behavioral therapy for primary insomnia. *American Journal of Psychiatry, 150*, 1259–1260.

Mimeault, V. & Morin, C.M. (1999). Self-help treatment for insomnia: Bibliotherapy with and without professional guidance. *Journal of Consulting and Clinical Psychology, 67*, 511–519.

Moldofsky, H. (1989). Sleep and fibrositis syndrome. *Rheumatoid Disorders Clinics of North America, 15*, 91–103.

Monroe, L.J. (1967). Psychological and physiological differences between good and poor sleepers. *Journal of Abnormal Psychology, 72*, 255–264.

Montplaisir, J. Nicolas, A., Godbout, R., & Walters, A. (2000). Restless legs syndrome and periodic limb movement disorder. In M. Kryger, T. Roth, & W. Dement (Eds.), *Principles and practice of sleep medicine* (3rd Ed., pp. 742–752). Philadelphia, Pa: W.B. Sauders.

Morin, C.M. (1993). *Insomnia: Psychological assessment and management.* New York: Guilford Press.

Morin, C.M. (1994). Dysfunctional beliefs and attitudes about sleep: Preliminary scale development and description. *The Behavior Therapist, 17*, 163–164.

Morin, C.M. (2001). Combined treatments of insomnia. In M.T. Sammons and N.B. Schmidt. *Combined treatments for mental disorders* (pp. 111–129). Washington, D.C.: American Psychological Association.

Morin, C.M., Bastien, C., Guay, B., Radouco-Thomas, M., Leblanc, J., & Vallières, A. (2003). Insomnia and chronic use of benzodiazepines: A randomized clinical trial of supervised tapering, cognitive-behavior therapy, and a combined approach to facilitate benzodiazepine discontinuation. Manuscript under review.

Morin, C.M., Blais, F., & Savard, J. (2002). Are changes in beliefs and attitudes about sleep related to sleep improvements in the treatment of insomnia? *Behaviour Research and Therapy, 40*, 741–752.

Morin, C.M., Colecchi, C.A., Ling, W.D., & Sood, R.K. (1995). Cognitive behavior therapy to facilitate benzodiazepine discontinuation among hypnotic-dependent patients with insomnia. *Behavior Therapy, 26*, 733–745.

Morin, C.M., Colecchi, C.A., Stone, J., Sood, R., & Brink, D. (1999). Behavioral and pharmacological therapies for late-life insomnia: A randomized clinical trial. *Journal of the American Medical Association, 281*, 991–999.

Morin, C.M., Gaulier, B., Barry, T., & Kowatch, R. (1992). Patients' acceptance of psychological and pharmacological therapies for insomnia. *Sleep, 15*, 302–305.

Morin, C.M., Hauri, P.J., Espie, C.A., Spielman, A.J., Buysse, D.J., & Bootzin, R.R. (1999). Nonpharmacological treatment of chronic insomnia. *Sleep, 22*, 1134–1156.

Morin, C.M., Rodrigue, S., & Ivers, H. (2003). The role of stress, arousal, and coping skills in primary insomnia. *Psychosomatic Medicine, 65*, 259–267.

Morin, C.M., Stone, J., Jones, S., & McDonald, K. (1994). Psychological treatment of insomnia: A clinical replication series with 100 patients. *Behavior Therapy, 25,* 291–309.

Morin, C.M., Stone, J., Trinkle, D., Mercer, J., & Remsberg, S. (1993). Dysfunctional beliefs and attitudes about sleep among older adults with and without insomnia complaints. *Psychology and Aging, 8,* 463–467.

Morris, M., Lack, L., & Dawson, D. (1990). Sleep-onset insomniacs have delayed temperature rhythms. *Sleep, 13,* 1–14.

National Institutes of Health. (1984). Consensus Conference. Drugs and insomnia. The use of medications to promote sleep. *Journal of the American Medical Association, 251,* 2410–2414.

National Institutes of Health. (1991). National Institutes of Health Consensus Development Conference Statement: The treatment of sleep disorders of older people. *Sleep, 14,* 169–177.

National Institutes of Health. (1996). NIH releases statement on behavioral and relaxation approaches for chronic pain and insomnia. *American Family Physician, 53,* 1877–1880.

Nicassio, P.M., Mendlowitz, D.R., Fussell, J.J., & Petras, L. (1985). The phenomenology of the pre-sleep state: The development of the pre-sleep arousal scale. *Behaviour Research and Therapy, 23,* 263–271.

Nowell, P.D., Mazumdar, S., Buysse, D.J., Dew, M.A., Reynolds, C.F., & Kupfer, D.J. (1997). Benzodiazepines and zolpidem for chronic insomnia: A meta- analysis of treatment efficacy. *Journal of the American Medical Association, 278,* 2170–2177.

O'Connor, K., Bélanger, L., Marchand, A., Dupuis, G., Élie, R., & Boyer, R. (1999). Psychological distress and adaptational problems associated with discontinuation of benzodiazepines. *Addictive Behavior, 24,* 537–541.

Otto, M.W., Pollack, M.H., Sachs, G.S., Reiter, S.R., Meltzer-Brody, S., & Rosenbaum, J.F. (1993). Discontinuation of benzodiazepine treatment: Efficacy of cognitive-behavioral therapy for patients with panic disorder. *American Journal of Psychiatry, 150,* 1485–1490.

Padesky, C.A. & Greenberger, D. (1995). *Mind over mood: Clinician's guide.* New York: Guilford Press.

Parrino, L. & Terzano, M.G. (1996). Polysomnographic effects of hypnotic drugs: A review. *Psychopharmacology, 126,* 1–16.

Perlis, M., Aloia, M., Millikan, A., Boehmler, J., Smith, M., Greenblatt, D., et al. (2000). Behavioral treatment of insomnia: A clinical case series study. *Journal of Behavioral Medicine, 23,* 149–161.

Perlis, M.L., Smith, M.T., Andrews P.J., Orff, H., & Giles, D.E. (2001). Beta/Gamma EEG activity in patients with primary and secondary insomnia and good sleeper controls. *Sleep, 24,* 110–117.

Prochaska, J.O., DiClemente, C.C., & Norcross, J.C. (1992). In search of how people change. Applications to addictive behaviors. *American Psychologist, 47,* 1102–1114.

Quesnel, C., Savard, J., Simard, S., Ivers, H., & Morin, C.M. (2003). Efficacy of cognitive-behavioral therapy for insomnia in women treated for non-metastatic breast cancer. *Journal of Consulting and Clinical Psychology, 71,* 189–200.

Reite, M., Buysse, D., Reynolds, C., & Mendelson, W. (1995). The use of polysomnography in the evaluation of insomnia. *Sleep, 18,* 58–70.

Reynolds, C.F., Taska, L.S., Sewitch, D.E., Restifo, K., Coble, P.A., & Kupfer, D.J. (1984). Persistent psychophysiologic insomnia: Preliminary research diagnostic criteria and EEG sleep data. *American Journal of Psychiatry, 141,* 804–805.

Rickels. K., Morris, R.J., Newman, H., Rosenfeld, H., Schiller, H., & Weinstock, R. (1983). Diphenhydramine in insomniac family practice patients: A double-blind study. *Journal of Clinical Pharmacology, 23,* 234–242.

Rickels, K., Case, W.G., Schweizer, E., Garcia-Espana, F., & Fridman, R. (1990). Benzodiazepine dependence: Management of discontinuation. *Psychopharmacology Bulletin, 26,* 63–68.

Riedel, B.W. & Lichstein, K.L. (2000). Insomnia and daytime functioning. *Sleep Medicine Reviews, 4,* 277–298.

Roehrs, T. (1993). Alcohol. In M.A., Carskadon, A. Rechtschaffen, G. Richardson, T. Roth, & J. Siegel (Eds.). *Encyclopedia of sleep and dreaming* (pp. 21–23). New York: MacMillan.

Roehrs, T. & Roth, T. (2000). Hypnotics: Efficacy and adverse effects. In M. Kryger, T. Roth, W. Dement (Eds.), *Principles and practice of sleep medicine* (3rd. Ed., pp. 414–418). Philadelphia, PA: W.B. Saunders.

Roy-Byrne, P.P., & Cowley, D.S. (Eds.). (1991). *Benzodiazepines in clinical practice: Risks and benefits.* Washington, DC: American Psychiatric Press.

Sadeh, A. Hauri, P.J., Kripke, D.F., & Lavie, P. (1995). The role of actigraphy in the evaluation of sleep disorders. *Sleep, 18,* 288–302.

Salin-Pascual, R.J., Roehrs T.A., Merlotti, L.A., Zorick, F., & Roth, T. (1992). Long-term study of the sleep of insomnia patients with sleep state misperception and other insomnia patients. *Sleep, 15,* 252–256.

Sateia, M.J., Doghramji, K., Hauri, P.J., & Morin, C.M. (2000). Evaluation of chronic insomnia. An American Academy of Sleep Medicine review. *Sleep, 23,* 243–308.

Savard, J. Laroche, L., Simard, S., Ivers, H., & Morin, C. M. (2003). Chronic insomnia and immune functioning. *Psychosomatic Medicine, 65,* 211–221.

Savard, J , Simard, S., Quesnel, C., Ivers, H., & Morin, C.M. (2002). Cognitive-behavior therapy for insomnia secondary to breast cancer. *Sleep, 25,* A72.

Schneider-Helmert, D. (1988). Why low-dose benzodiazepine-dependent insomniacs can't escape their sleeping pills. *Acta Psychiatrica Scandinavica, 78,* 706–711.

Schweizer, E., Rickels, K., Case, W.G., & Greenblatt, D.J. (1990). Long-term therapeutic use of benzodiazepines: II. Effects of gradual taper. *Archives of General Psychiatry, 47,* 908–915.

Smith, M.T., Perlis, M.L., Park, A., Smith, M.S., Pennington, J., Giles, D.E., et al. (2002). Comparative meta-analysis of pharmacotherapy and behavior therapy for persistent insomnia. *American Journal of Psychiatry, 159,* 5–11.

Soldatos, C.R., Dikeos, D.G., & Whitehead, A. (1999). Tolerance and rebound insomnia with rapidly eliminated hypnotics: A meta-analysis of sleep laboratory studies. *International Clinics of Psychopharmacology, 14,* 287–303.

Spielman, A.J. & Anderson, M.W. (1999). The clinical interview and treatment planning as a guide to understanding the nature of insomnia: The CCNY Interview for Insomnia (pp. 385–426). In S. Chokroverty (Eds). *Sleep disorders medicine: basic science, technical considerations and clinical aspects (2nd Edition)*. Boston: Butterworth-Heinemann.

Spielman, A.J. & Glovinsky, P.B. (1991). The varied nature of insomnia (pp. 1–15). In P. Hauri (Ed). *Case studies in insomnia*. New York: Plenum Press.

Spielman, A.J., Saskin, P., & Thorpy, M.J. (1987). Treatment of chronic insomnia by restriction of time in bed. *Sleep, 10*, 45–56.

Stepanski, E., Zorich, F., Roehrs, T.A., Young, D., & Roth, T. (1988). Daytime alertness in patients with chronic insomnia compared with asymptomatic control subjects. *Sleep, 11*, 54–60.

Stepanski, E., Zorick, F., & Roth, T. (1991). Pharmacotherapy of insomnia. In P.J. Hauri (Ed.), *Case studies in insomnia* (pp. 115–129). New York: Plenum press.

Stevenson, C. & Ernst, E. (2000). Valerian for insomnia: A systematic review of randomized clinical trials. *Sleep Medicine, 1*, 91–99.

Vallières, A. (2002). *Le traitement séquentiel de l'insomnie [Sequential treatment of insomnia]*. Unpublished doctoral dissertation. Université Laval, Québec.

Van Egeren, L., Haynes, S.N., Franzen, M., & Hamilton, J. (1983). Presleep cognitions and attributions in sleep-onset insomnia. *Journal of Behavioral Medicine, 6*, 217–232.

Vignola, A., Lamoureux, C., Bastien, C.H., & Morin, C.M. (2000). Effects of chronic insomnia and use of benzodiazepines on daytime performance in older adults. *Journal of Gerontology, 55*, P54–P62.

Vollrath, M., Wicki, W., & Angst, J. (1989). The Zurich study. VIII: Insomnia: Association with depression, anxiety, somatic syndromes, and course of insomnia. *European Archives of Psychiatry and Neurological Sciences, 239*, 113–124.

Wagner, J., Wagner, M.L., & Hening, W. (1998). Beyond benzodiazepines: Alternative pharmacologic agents for the treatment of insomnia. *The Annals of Pharmacotherapy, 32*, 680–691.

Walters, A.S., Hickey, K., Maltzman, J., Verrico, T., Joseph, D., Hening, W., et al. (1996). A questionnaire study of 138 patients with restless legs syndrome: The 'Night-Walkers' survey. *Neurology, 46*, 92–95.

Watts, F.N., East, M.P., & Coyle, K. (1995). Insomniacs' perceived lack of control over sleep. *Psychology and Health, 10*, 81–95.

Whitney, C.W., Enright, P.L., Newman, A.B., Bonekat, W., Foley, D., & Quan, S.F. (1998). Correlates of daytime sleepiness in 4,578 elderly persons: The cardiovascular health study. *Sleep, 21*, 27–36.

Wicklow, A. & Espie, C.A. (2000). Intrusive thoughts and their relationship to actigraphic measurement of sleep: towards a cognitive model of insomnia. *Behaviour Research & Therapy, 38*, 679–693.

Wohlgemuth, W.K. & Edinger, J.D. (2000). Sleep restriction therapy. In K.L. Lichstein & C.M. Morin (Eds.).*Treatment of late-life insomnia* (pp. 147–166). Thousand Oaks, Ca.: Sage Publications.

Index